AUTISM
A Complex Learning Disorder

A MULTIDISCIPLINARY PERSPECTIVE

Dr. S. Ramaa
Regional Institute of Education (NCERT)
Mysore 570006, India

Regency Publications
New Delhi 110 008

Division of
DAYA PUBLISHING HOUSE
4760-61/23, Ansari Road,
Darya Ganj, New Delhi - 110 002
Phone: 23245578, 23244987; Fax: (011) 23260116
E-mail: info@regency-books.com
Website: www.regencybooks.com

ISBN 81-86030-62-X

Published by Regency Publications, 20/36-G, Old Market, West Patel Nagar, New Delhi 110 008 and printed at Radiant Printers, New Delhi, Phones: 574 0038, 571 2539; Telefax: 578 3571.

Preface

The book is prepared as a part of my post-doctoral work at University of Manchester, UK.

In the book autism is considered as a complex learning disorder in contrast to general learning disorder (mental retardation and specific learning disorders (like dyslexia, dyscalculia, etc.). In order to help children with autism, a multidisciplinary approach is essential. Usually autism is viewed from different disciplinary points of view in isolation. But for planning and executing intervention there is a need to understand from multidisciplinary perspective. The specialists from the field of psychiatry, paediatrics, clinical psychology, special education, speech and language therapy, physiotherapy should plan well coordinated programme for helping them.

As a basis for planning the intervention programmes there is a need to make a thorough review of the research conducted in the area of autism, particularly in the recent years. In this book such an attempt has been made.

The research work related to autism is based on certain theoretical assumptions. These theories can be broadly classified into four areas: Biological, Neuro-physiological, Psychophysiological and Psychological. The important assumptions of each of these theories and the research work carried out under these theoretical backgrounds are described in detail. A selective synthesis of the theoretical assumptions as well as research findings are made in order to obtain a more comprehensive and adequate picture of autism. Implications for intervention are also suggested. Certain hypotheses are also formulated for future course of action.

The manuscript was reviewed by my experts both in England and India and they gave valuable and pertinent suggestions. Suitable modifications were made in the manuscript based on their suggestions. I hope the personnel from different disciplines who are concerned with autism will be benefitted by reading this book.

22.12.1997 **S. Ramaa**

Acknowledgements

I express my heartfelt thanks to the following persons for their help in preparing and publishing this book:

Prof. Peter L. Mittler, Former Director and Dean, School of Education, University of Manchester, Manchester, U.K.

Dr. Shoba Srinath, Additional Professor, Department of Psychiatry, National Institute of Mental Health and Neuro Sciences, Bangalore.

Prof. P.R. Nayar, Former Dean and Head, Department of Education, Manasagangothri, Mysore.

Mr. Vijay Naidu, my husband, Executive Trustee and President, United Earth Peace Academy, Mysore.

The Publisher, Regency Publications, New Delhi

S. RAMAA

Contents

CHAPTER 1

Autism: Diagnostic Criteria and Specific Difficulties in Different Aspects of Development

1.1 Introduction

Autism is a perplexing life-long mental handicap. Autism is a wide umbrella term. Children with autism have different levels of intelligence. However all of them share certain common characteristics.

The 10th revision of the World Health Organization's International Classification of Diseases and Related Health Problems (ICD-10), 1992 and the American Psychiatric Association's Diagnostic Statistical Manuals DSM-III (1980), DSM-IIIR (1987) and DSM-IV (1994) included autism under Pervasive Developmental Disorders. In DSM-IIIR Pervasive Developmental Disorders are treated as a subcategory under — Developmental Disorders whereas in DSM-IV (1994) they are included under the majority category — Disorders of Psychological Development. Pervasive Developmental Disorders imply deviance rather than delay in development, although they involve some degree of delay (DSM-IV, 1994).

1.2 Diagnostic Criteria for Autism

Nearly 75% of autistics have mental retardation of different degrees. It is difficult to distinguish a child with autism and mental retardation, from a mentally retarded child who is not autistic. Certain sets of criteria are essential for diagnosing autism. Four main sets of diagnostic criteria are specified by ICD-9 and 10 (WHO, 1978 and 1987), DSM-III, DSM-IIIR (APA, 1980 and 1987). Rutter (1987) has made these criteria and descriptions further more explicit and clear. They are given below.

Onset Before 3 Years of Age

Occasional cases of autistic like disorders do occur after the age of 3, but they are rare and usually due to acquired brain disease or genetic disorders of later manifestation — such as the cerebral lipoidoses.

Deviance in the Development of Social Relations

More specifically,

a. failure to use eye-to-eye gaze, facial expression, body posture, and gesture to regulate social interaction;
b. rarely seeking others for comfort or affection;
c. rarely initiating comfort to others or responding to other people's distress or happiness;
d. rarely initiating interactive play with others;
e. rarely greeting others; and
f. no peer friendships in terms of sharing of interests, activities, and emotions — despite ample opportunities. (In each case, these have to be considered in relation to mental age.)

Abnormalities in Communication

These features include:

a. delay in, or total lack of development of spoken language that is not compensated for by use of gesture or mime as alternative modes of communication (often preceded by a lack of communicative babbling);
b. failure to respond to the communication of others, such as (when young) not responding when called by name;
c. relative failure to initiate or sustain conversational interchange in which there is a to and fro responsivity to the communication of other person;
d. stereotyped and repetitive use of language;
e. use of you when I is meant;

f. idiosyncratic use of words;
g. abnormalities in pitch, stress, rate, rhythm, and intonation of speech;
h. lack of creativity and spontaneity not only in the use of social language but also in the preverbal skills; and
i. lack of varied/spontaneous "make-believe" play.

Restricted, Repetitive and Stereotyped Patterns of Behaviour

They include:
a. an encompassing pre-occupation with stereotyped and restricted patterns of interest;
b. attachment to unusual objects;
c. compulsive rituals;
d. stereotyped and repetitive motor mannerisms;
e. pre-occupations with part objects or non-functional elements of play materials; and
f. distress over changes in small details of the environment.

It is interesting to note that the criteria and sub-criteria are all observable and specific behavioural symptoms. No single clinical symptom is considered for diagnosis. There are different clinical types of mental retardation, different types of cerebral palsy, varied types of mental disorders, different kinds of learning disabilities. Autism seems to be different from the above kinds of disabilities in the sense that it is not possible to identify clear-cut subtypes within this major category of handicap. DSM-III-R (APA, 1987 — cited in Gillberg, 1990) suggests that out of the 16 symptoms suggested in the document at least 8 should be fulfilled, in order to treat a child as autistic. This implies that autistic children can have the above mentioned symptoms in any combination which results in a lot of heterogeneity among them, which in turn makes it extremely difficult to categorise them into different sub-groups.

Gillberg (1990), argues that it is not appropriate to distinguish "infantile autism" from the umbrella concept of "autistic spectrum disorders". His important arguments are:

- As evidenced in the Wing studies (Wing and Gould, 1979) though it is possible to identify "Kanner autism" from among the wider group of cases, they do not have a unifying biological or psychosocial background;

- Children with autistic behaviour with and without demonstrable neurological dysfunction do not differ from the behavioural point of view;
- Even among high level autism cases which comply clearly with the clinical descriptions provided by Kanner (1943), diverse conditions such as tuberous sclerosis and the fragile X chromosomal abnormality can be noticed (Gillberg et al., 1987); and
- There is considerable overlap between "typical" Kanner autism cases and cases now diagnosed as suffering from Asperger Syndrome (Wing, 1981; Gillberg, 1989).

However, Gillberg (1990) thinks that the notion of Asperger Syndrome — or "high level autism" — is important. Gillberg and Gillberg (1989) suggest the following characteristic features for Asperger Syndrome:

- severe impairment in reciprocal social interaction;
- all-absorbing, circumscribed interest;
- imposition of routine or interest;
- speech and language problems in spite of superficially excellent expressive language skills;
- non-verbal communication problems; and
- motor clumsiness.

According to Gillberg (1990) the concept of Asperger syndrome is important mainly because such disorders are much more common than as believed previously. However, unlike the case of typical autism they do not often lead to psychiatric consultation until adulthood. The need for psychiatric intervention is realised when it gets superimposed with problems such as depression, paranoid symptoms, confusion (under stress) and suicidal attempts (Tantam, 1988). This implies that psychiatrists dealing with adult patients need to be competent in diagnosing and handling autism spectrum disorders, including Asperger syndrome (Gillberg, 1990).

From the discussion above it seems that autism has four dimensions: Social Indifference, Communication Problems and Deviant "Personality Traits" as three symptomatic dimensions and Age of onset (Course of development) as the fourth dimension. The picture of autism seems to be more or less complete with all these four dimensions. The absence of any one of these aspects may give a diagnostic picture which is different from autism. Any how it appears very strange to notice that while conceptualising autism, the Sensory Deviation which is so obvious among them is neither taken into consideration nor made explicit.

Sensory Deviation refers to the following unusual responses to sensory stimuli (Wing and Wing, 1965; cited in Mittler, 1968):

Vision

- Inability to recognise things seen, mainly because of pronounced difficulty in differentiating figure from the ground.
- Use of peripheral vision, resulting in difficulty to recognise stationary objects, while readily recognising moving objects/ organisms.
- Visual avoidance.
- Some visual stimuli are sought after.

Hearing

- Apparent non-reaction to noise is typical at some stage. May fail to react to a loud noise behind but responds to rustle of a thin paper.
- Special interest in certain noises, like echoes, tapping, the noise of a flywheel, etc. Music is particularly enjoyed.
- Auditory avoidance is common, particularly to loud noises or to speech.

Other Senses

- Indifference to pain, cold, etc.
- Inability to localise a sensation.
- Unusual tastes or interests in unusual smells.
- Identify objects through licking, tapping, etc. rather than through sight or hearing.

In fact these appear to be more fundamental and relatively persistent problems among autistics. So it is highly essential to include them along with the salient characteristics of autism. In that case autism is not a "triad syndrome" as usually referred to but a "tetroid syndrome".

There appears to be a high correlation between various symptoms falling under each major criterion and also between those of other criteria which are thought to be the cardinal features of autism. However, one should be very careful in understanding the nature of such a relationship, as correlation need not necessarily imply causation on the one hand or a circular reaction on the other hand. This suggests the following:

— The various symptoms can exist relatively independent of each other to a certain extent; thus there is scope for quantitative variation as far as the extent of occurance of the particular symptoms are concerned.
— There can be a greater degree of mutual influence among the various symptoms of autism.
— The above two factors, in addition to the level of "global intelligence" are responsible in making a particular child relatively more autistic or less autistic at any stage of development and across the course of development.
— Therefore an attempt should be made to understand and explain each symptom or each set of symptoms separately and also in relation to other symptoms.

1.3 Specific Difficulties Experienced by Children with Autism

The knowledge of specific difficulties experienced by individuals with autism is helpful in planning intervention program for them. The Association of Head Teachers of Autistic Children and Adults (1985), UK, has described the specific difficulties of children with autism in detail.

Impaired Relationships and Self Image

a) Lack of self image

— Suffers a lack of personal identity and an impairment of his own self image.
— He is "asocial" tending to remain isolated, occupying himself with his own obsessional or ritualistic activity, and having an impaired sense of his own appropriate personal territory.

— Being unaware of himself, his actions and his effect on others, he is likely to display a lack of inhibition in his general behaviour.

b) Difficulty in relating to other people

— Impairment of the awareness of other people and their needs.
— An inappropriate social response to, and communication with others.
— An impairment of the ability to recognise human characteristics.

c) Difficulty in perception of meaningful relationships

— Impaired ability to see sequences of growth, time, action, etc.
— Impaired ability to see similarities or differences, like and unlike.
— Impaired ability to see a whole picture or a whole anything.
— Impaired ability to relate properties, eg. fire will burn.
— Impaired ability to generalise or transfer learning.
— Lack of awareness of the reality of what cannot be seen, and an impaired ability to separate reality from fantasy.
— Impaired awareness of the relationship of objects to each other, to themselves, and to other people, eg. as seen in an inability to comprehend the use of prepositions.
— Lack of judgment.
— Inability to be selective in the processing of information.

d) Difficulty in relating to outside stimuli

— Impairment of motivation lacking the desire to learn new skills and the desire to please.
— Impairment of the sense of touch, smell, taste.
— Impairment of the use of sight where he may be fascinated by visual stimuli such as lights or bright objects, and be uninterested in the rest of his environment.
— Inappropriate reaction to sounds.
— Inappropriate emotional response.
— Lack of awareness of real danger and a phobic response to harmless objects.

— Lack of awareness of cause and effect.
— Inappropriate reaction to change.

Deficiency in Adoptive Behaviours

a. Ritualistic, compulsive, obsessional behaviours.
b. Extreme irrational fears or phobias.
c. Rigidity of thought and action — This manifests itself in pre-occupation with sameness and difficulty with change.
d. Poor perception of reality — There is often confusion between inner and outer worlds.
e. Extreme Anxiety States, or "High Arousal".

Impaired Language and Communication Skills

Cognitive skills

a. Difficulty in language.
b. Patchy development of skills — No normal development of cognitive skills. Having a particular skill does not imply that 'earlier' skills will be present.
c. Specific difficulties in problem solving.
d. Play may be stuck at early stages of development.
e. Tend to have poor imitation skills.
f. Difficulty in directing attention to certain meaningful features of the environment.
g. Motivation and self-directed action are often lacking.
h. Time and causality are difficulty ideas to autistic children.
i. Poor sequencing ability.

Deficiency in perceptual-motor skills

— Lack of body awareness, body control and perceptual control.

As implied in the specific difficulties discussed above, autism is a complex learning disorder. In order to help children with autism a multidisciplinary approach is essential. The specialists from the field of psychiatry, paediatrics, clinical psychology, special education, physiotherapy, speech and language therapy should plan a well coordinated programme for helping them. Autism is viewed from different disciplinary point of view in isolation. But for planning and executing intervention programme there is a need to understand autism from multidisciplinary perspective. Hence an attempt has been made in the following chapters to discuss the important findings of recent research work in the area of autism. These research works are based on certain theoretical assumptions. Therefore these research findings are discussed under different theoretical perspectives.

CHAPTER 2

Biogenic Theories of Autism

2.1 Introduction

It seems meaningful to classify the theories of autism broadly into the following categories:

Theories of Autism

- Biological
- Neuro Physiological
- Psycho-Physiological
- Psychological

Though the above classification is mainly from the point of view of convenience for discussion, it is based on certain key features like the angle from which attempt has been made to explain autism, the extent of direct relationship permissible between the behavioural symptoms of autism and the factors hypothesised to be responsible for such features, the techniques employed to verify such hypotheses, as well as the possible implications for the intervention of autism.

2.2 Biogenic Theories

The biogenic theories of autism include mainly genetic basis theory as well as abnormality in the anatomy of the neurobiological system and these are discussed below.

2.2.1 *The Genetic Basis of Autism*

In fact genetic basis theory is the oldest theory of autism. Kanner (1943) himself states: "We must assume that these children have come into the world with innate inability to form the usual biologically provided affective contact with people, just as other children come into the world with innate physical or intellectual handicaps". This statement implies the following:

- Kanner was more concerned with the inability of the autistics to develop affective contact with others rather than their cognitive deficits.
- He attributed such an inability to an inborn defect or abnormality.

Like Kanner even Asperger (cited in Uta Frith, 1989) suggested independently that there is a "disturbance of contact" at some deep level of affect and/or instinct.

While discussing about the genetic basis of autism Rutter (1968) comments that in the quarter of the century since Kanner many other writers discussed autism in relation to a basic constitutional defect or abnormality; some investigators like Rimland (1965) have suggested that this defect may be genetically determined. However, Rutter (1968) was of the opinion that there is no sufficient data to support the possibility of a genetic basis of autism, as the rate of autism among siblings is very low for a hereditary disorder (Rutter, 1967). He has suggested that twin studies should be helpful in determining whether autism has a genetic basis or not. Finally, he has concluded that the available data by no means rules out the possibility of a genetic basis and also it does not provide any support for such a hypothesis.

Rutter (1967) expressed doubt regarding the possibility of a chromosomal anomaly as a causative factor for autism as the maternal age is normal (Creak and Ini, 1960; Lotter, 1967) in the case of autistics. However, in recent years it has been proved beyond chance factors that fragile-X syndrome is strongly associated with autism (Wahlstrom, Gillberg, Gustavson and Holmgren, 1986) and it is now considered one of the major underlying dysfunctions in a substantial proportion of cases with autism (Gillberg, Ohlson et al.). Concomitant autism-fragile-X has been reported to occur mainly in boys, but in 1986 a study on a pair of monozygotic female twins with autism and the fragile-X syndrome (AFRAX) was reported indicating this condition is not exclusive to males (Gillberg, Ohlson et al., 1988).

The physical and psychological characteristics noticed among those affected with fragile-X are neither distinct nor unique to them. August and Lockhart, in 1984 and De La Cruz, in 1985, reported that among males they noticed the following characteristics:

- Tend to have a long narrow face with a high forehead and long low set ears.
- Have a high arched palate.
- Show poor muscle tone with delay in fine and gross motor development.
- After puberty have larger sex organs.

The study on monozygotic female twins of chronological age 7.8 years with AFRAX, as reported and discussed in Gillberg, Ohlson et al. (1988) reveals that they exhibited the following characteristics:

- Slight mongoloid slant of eyelids
- Big ears
- Adherent ear-lobes
- Thin feet
- Squint
- Slight sight problem (but refuse to wear glasses)
- "Fussy hair"
- Percentage of fragile-X-positive cells — 24% and 46%. (Authors' Notes — They look normal in spite of minor physical deviances. They are and have always been physically healthy.)

Their head circumference, length, weight were identical. Epilepsy was absent in both the cases. The child with 46% of fragile-X cells was observed to be a little more behaviourally disturbed and somewhat more mentally retarded than the other.

The authors infer that as both parents appear to be chromosomally normal the abnormality noticed among these girls nrepresents a new mutation or that the parents do not express the fragile site. Further they remark that the twins did not show any typical physical features suggestive of the fragile-X syndrome. However, they conclude that it is clear now that the fragile-X chromosome abnormality is sometimes associated with learning disorders and even mental retardation in girls. They recommend the need to examine the chromosomes of autistic girls in a folic acid-depleted-medium.

Fragile-X was only discovered when the medium used to culture chromosomes was deficient in folic acid — that is, in the presence of folic acid the chromosomes do not appear fragile or broken, which led to the speculation that administration of folic acid might 'repair' the chromosomes and improve general functioning (Clements, 1987). The studies which were independently conducted by Lejeune (1982) and Gustavson et al. (1985) clearly indicated a positive effect from administration of folic acid in terms of improvement in autistic-like behaviours. Further, the study by Gustavson revealed that there was no improvement in the overall level of intellectual functioning. This finding was confirmed in a controlled folic acid and placebo trial (Carpenter et al., 1983). From the findings of these studies Clements (1987) conclude that oral administration of folic acid does lead to marked reduction or complete elimination of chromosome fragility. He is hopeful that if screening for fragile-X became a part of routine diagnostic procedures then an early intervention programme with combination of folic acid treatment and intensive work on language and social skills might yield important results in terms of behavioural adjustment and level of functioning.

The hypothesis relating to the genetic basis of autism appears to be still shaky. This is mainly because of the two reasons stated below (vide Rutter, 1967).

Firstly, the chances to conduct the follow-up studies with the intention to find out whether the children of autistics are going to be autistics are extremely less, as autistics rarely marry and have children.

Secondly the number of twin studies are less as autistic twins are very rare.

In such a condition, it seems, one of the alternative techniques could be to study the egg cells and sperms in the case of autistic females and males respectively. If there is any significant variation in them that may suggest the possible genetic basis. In order to further confirm whether those variations would lead to autistic syndrome, comparative studies could be undertaken. For eg. studying the gamets/sex cells, among autistics, Down syndromes and other mental handicaps wherein there is an establishment of genetic causation like phenyl ketenuria, galactosemia, etc. Though it is not a final test, as phenotype may be still different from genotype, studies of this sort may provide certain valid clues.

2.2.2 *Abnormalities in the Neurobiological System*

Like genetic basis of autism, autism was also thought to be attributable to brain damage by some investigators. Rutter (1967) has very precisely suggested the main evidences in favour of brain damage hypothesis. They are as follows:

1. A clinical picture which is indistinguishable from infantile autism may develop after overt brain disease such as encephalitis when it occurs in infancy or early childhood.
2. Autistic children who have no abnormalities which are detectable on a neurological examination in early or middle childhood, may later develop evidence of organic brain dysfunction. In particular, epileptic fits develop in adolescence in upto one sixth of cases.
3. While the frequent occurance of cognitive, language, and perceptual defects does not in itself necessarily indicate structural pathology of the brain, their presence is suggestive of some kind of organic brain dysfunction.

According to Rutter (1967), the following are the main arguments against brain damage as a general explanation for autism:

1. There is no evidence of brain damage in at least half the cases of autism.
2. The types of brain damage found in association with autism are all types more usually found in association with non-autistic conditions; we are still left with the question why brain damage leads to autism in a few children, but not in others who, apparently, have the same kind of brain damage (Bettelheim, 1967).

Rutter (1967) was of the opinion that much of the evidence which could be crucial is still missing; there are no published histopathological studies, the E.E.G. studies in the literature are inadequate and contradictory, and metabolic investigations are still in their infancy. Moreover, the tools to measure brain function are still very inadequate.

Twenty years after Rutter's criticisms mentioned above, now there are promising techniques available to make a detailed study of the anatomy of the nervous system. Magnetic resonance tomography or Magnetic resonance imaging (MRI) which is a relatively new method is one such technique.

Very few studies have so far been performed on the classic syndrome of autism with the aid of magnetic resonance imaging (Ekman et al., 1989). Ekman et al. (1989) and Gillberg (1990) have summarised the findings of those studies. The important findings are as follows:

— Hypoplasia of cerebellar vermal lobules 6 and 7 in 14 out of 18 autistics who were relatively high functioning versus 12 normal controls (Courchesne et al., 1988).
— Brainstem (in particular the pons) significantly smaller in a group of 13 relatively high functioning autistic persons in comparison with 35 "medical" age matched controls; same group demonstrated widening of fourth ventricle (Gaffney et al., 1988 Gaffney and Tsai, 1987).
— Widening of fourth ventricle in "high functioning" children with autism (Herold et al., 1987).
— Significant and unusual cerebellar malformation, hypoplasia in the posterior vermis and hypoplasia of the medial aspect of each cerebellar hemisphere; pathology in the right posterior cerebral hemisphere in the case of a 21 year old autistic man with normal IQ (Courchesne et al., 1987).
— Clinically detectable lesions including heterotopic grey matter, basal ganglia abnormalities, and dilated lateral and fourth ventricles in 6 out of 14 high functioning autistics (Gaffney and Tsai, 1987).
— The cisterna magna (a room located between the cerebellum and the posterior fossa, filled with cerebrospinal fluid) was wide in one out of 15 cases and the arteria basilaris (an artery located in the sulcus basilaris pontis, which gives away branches to the cerebellum and a small branch to the inner ear and the pons) was large in another patient. In four cases a varying degree of asymmetry between the brain hemispheres was present (Ekman et al., 1989).

In some studies autopsy was done to find out whether there are any structural changes in the central nervous system among autistics. The autopsy of a 29 year old man with clear autism showed major cellular and structural changes in hippocampus, amygdala and cerebellum including Purkinje cell loss (Baumann and Kemper, 1985). The autopsy of four autistics by Ritvo et al. (1986), clearly showed Purkinje cell loss in the cerebellum of all of them.

On the basis of the above findings, different authors formulated different hypotheses as the possible major causes of autism. Courchesne et al. (1988), propose that autism is strongly associated with abnormalities in the neocerebellar vermal parts of the cerebellum, representing a developmental hypoplasia. According to them the neocerebellar maldevelopment could potentially affect cognitive development and behaviour control in either a direct way or by way of connections from the neocerebellum to the brain stem and the hypothalamus. Reiss (1988) also thinks that autistic symptomatology may arise due to damage to the vermis during critical periods.

Gillberg (1990), has noticed that the most consistent recent finding of all in the study of neurobiology has been associated with brainstem pathology — enlarged fourth ventricle. Prolongation of brainstem transmission time (Ornitz, 1985), and association of hydrocephalus and damage to brainstem nerve nuclei (Moebius syndrome) with autism (Fernel, Gillberg and Wendt, 1990; Gillberg and Steffenburg, 1989) - all suggest to the level of brainstem pathophysiology in autism (Gillberg, 1990). However he appreciates the statement made by Tanguay and Edwards in 1982, that whatever defects are noticed among older patients may only be "the whisper of the bang" and higher brain centres might have been rendered dysfunctional by the damage at the brainstem level. According to him the indirect support for such a developmental neural theory could also be found in the studies which suggest that abnormal sensory responses are most typical of infancy (Dahlgren and Gillberg, 1989; Ornitz, 1989), whereas a variety of social defects are characteristics of the preschool years.

Ekman et al. (1989), have recommended that planimetrical, quantitative studies of the size of the fourth ventricle, the cerebral halves, and the cerebellum, and comparison of these results with a matched control group are required to further clarify the matter. However, they infer that the seemingly contradictory results of the investigations of the autistics could assert the fact that autism is the result of several different causes, acting through some common pathways to produce the symptoms of the syndrome.

If the assumptions made by Ekman et al. (1989) are valid then it seems more fruitful to make attempts to find out those common pathways in order to establish the causal relationships between biological defects and autistic syndrome. That should be an objective for future studies in this line, as ultimately the findings of such studies are the ones which would help in providing different kinds of intervention, particularly psychological and educational interventions.

CHAPTER 3

Neuro-physiological Theories

3.1 Introduction

The hypotheses relating to variation in neurophysiology as cause for autism are diverse in nature. It is quite interesting to review the assumptions which are basic to these hypotheses, kinds of studies conducted in order to verify them, the results obtained and also the suggested implications. In the following paragraphs a detailed account of the theories which fall under the umbrella term "Neurophysiology" are given.

3.2 Unusual Immune Response Among Autistics

There are studies which point out that autistic individuals may have a changed immune response. The theoretical issues related to immune system, as well as the studies which attempted to study the immune responses among autistics are discussed in detail by Rowell (1989).

The immune response system has evolved to protect the individual from the harmful effects created within the body due to presence of non-self materials like, viruses, bacteria and other microorganisms, and blood from other animals or individuals. The immune response operates at the molecular level as a particular cell is identified as a self or non-self on the basis of presence or absence of certain specific groups of molecules on the surface of that cell. The molecular identification marker flags are known as antigenic determinants, and the foreign materials which induce the operation of the immune system in response to their presence are known as antigens (Rowell, 1989).

In rare cases the body considers its self-flag as foreigner antigen. As a result the immune response is activated and antibodies are produced which attack the body's own cells. This process is known as an auto-immune response and the antibodies thus produced as autoantibodies (Rowell, 1989).

The autoantibodies, are capable of crossing the placenta and brain blood barrier and of acting on the developing foetus for a period several weeks after the birth of the baby.

On the basis of the observations made in studies related to immune systems of autistic children (Stubbs, 1976; Warren and his coworkers, 1986; Stubbs and his coworkers, 1978 and 1984; Markowitz, 1983; Weizman and his coworkers, 1982; Todd and Ciaranello, 1985; Stubbs, 1988; and Rowell, 1988) concluded that an altered immune response may be present in autistics. The finding that autistic children did not exhibit immune response when rubella virus was induced to their body could establish link between a prenatal exposure to an antigen, the rubella virus, and the development of the autistic syndrome due to brain damage in the developing foetus or due to a damaging foreign material, cell or virus to which the child has no immune defence. Tissue damage resulting from foreign materials or their toxins in turn precipitate the onset of an autoimmune response. Further Rowell (1989), suggests that the exact nature of the antigens involved in the initiation of the response,whether bacterial, viral or other materials such as food or the environment, and the time at which exposure occurs, whether pre- or postnatal, and even if the changes observed are a cause of or consequence of autism, all need to be explored in future research in this direction.

3.3 Metabolic Error as an Explanation for Autism

Increased levels of urinary bioactive peptides (compounds formed by the union of two or more aminoacids) were observed among autistics by Reichelt et al. (1981) and Reichelt et al. (1986) and confirmed by Israngun et al. (1986).

According to Reichlet there are three types of autistic syndromes (Reichlet et al., 1986), the salient features of which are as follows:

Type A

— Typically starts after a period of normal development;
— Shows increased galvanic skin conductance fluctuations;
— Very high levels of spontaneous fluctuations and very poor habituation to sensory stimuli.

Type B1

— Characterised by neonatal onset of hypotonia, which gradually worsens;
— The autistic symptoms are less dominant and often show a more panencephalic picture without known cause (i.e. no infective etiology).

Type B2

— Present from the early neonatal period onwards;
— Shows increased skin conductance, on average, lower than Type A;
— Exhibits poor sensory habituation.

On the basis of observation made by Shattock (1988), that parents of autistics stress alimentary problems among their children, Reichelt et al. (1989) attributed Type A to gluten (constituent of wheat flour and protein in nature; responsible for the malabsorption syndrome), Type B2 to milk derived exorphins and phosphorylated peptides, and Type B1 to both.

With the above hypotheses in mind they attempted to treat 15 patients with autistic syndromes, through gluten-free/gluten-reduced and milk-free/milk-reduced diets for a period of more than one year.

The treatment yielded the following results (Reichelt, 1989):

- Unexpectedly the frequency of epileptic fits decreased drastically on diet, and altogether disappeared in one case.
- Clear cut abstinence problems with skin rashes, itching, and various autonomic phenomena.

From the above findings the investigators concluded that the autistic syndromes may be the result of a genetic peptidase deficiency, which causes peptide accumulation and further peptidase inhibition. Further they suggested that the peptide overload is mainly of dietary origin. They also recommended that the treatment for the autistic syndromes should be dietary; however, dietary treatment can only make the autistic ready for psychological/behavioural treatment, and not actually replace this kind of treatment.

3.4 Dysfunction of Opioid System in Autism

The theoretical and empirical bases for a hypothesis that opioid excess may be one of the important or even the single most causative factor for autistic syndrome has been discussed in greater depth by Pankseep and Lensing in 1989. Opioids are endogenously-produced chemical substances which have multiple functions. A few important functions are analgesic, neuro-behavioural and hormonal. The basic assumptions of such a theory of autism as well as the evidence available in favour of those assumptions are highlighted below (Panskeep and Lensing, 1989).

Although it is very difficult to attribute the bewildering array of symptoms exhibited by autistics to a unitary psychoneural dysfunction, there is a greater agreement that the failure to exhibit appropriate social responsivity and psychosocial development may lie at the very core of the brain disorder. If social motivation arises from hard-wired emotional systems of the brain, then the neurobiological dysfunction of such children may be conceptually more straightforward than the diversity of outward symptoms would suggest. As autistic children have a low desire for companionship, many of their eventually cognitive deficits may be secondary to their failure to learn social norms and cultural knowledge. If social-affective deficits are in fact the primary deficit in autistic disorders, then identification of the underlying neural dysfunctions of autism may depend on our understanding of brain mechanisms which mediate social emotions. Though the neuroscientific work in this direction is still immature, recently it has been recognised that the desire for social interaction may arise unconditionally from genetically determined brain circuits which make social interactions emotionally desirable.

It is but natural for a mammal to be a socially dependent animal. Survival and normal development among mammals are premised on the ability of the young to perceive a need for social companionship and to establish firm attachment bonds with adults capable of providing nurturance and care. It is now certain that social interaction is desirable and social isolation highly aversive. From this it follows that concrete knowledge concerning the nature of brain circuits which mediate separation distress and social rewards can generate specific testable hypotheses relating to the cause and symptoms of autism. If social circuits which mediate social intent are constitutionally unresponsive, such a condition may be due to any of the following reasons:

- Inadequate development of neural elements within such circuits during brain growth;
- Deranged synaptic connectives or chemistries.

As specific neuropharmacological tools are available the last possibility is certainly the most hopeful and beneficial from the therapeutic perspective. The hypothesis formulated by Pankseep (1979 & 1981), Panskeep and Sahley (1987), Sahley and Pankseep (1987), is that excessive brain opioid activity may constitutionally inhibit social motivation, resulting in autistic isolation and aloofness.

The key lines of behavioural brain research which can throw much light on the underlying nature of autism are (Pankseep and Lensing, 1989):

1. study of the neurobiological nature of brain circuits which mediate the emotional distress arising from social isolation,
2. study of brain mechanisms which mediate social bonding (which provide the discriminative mechanisms for identifying especially important social companions such as friends, parents and others willing to share important social and economic resources), and,
3. identification of brain mechanisms which precipitate rough-and-tumble juvenile play (which may be the primal way in which social engagement/interaction strategies are learnt).

Pankseep and Lensing (1989), believe that the most important lines of evidence for understanding the neurobiological nature of social intent will be derived from the study of separation-distress/social-reward systems which presumably inform animals, especially young and relatively helpless ones, of their momentary "connectedness" to other animals capable and willing to provide nurturance, protection and support. They assume that from a theoretical perspective, any neurochemical influence which extinguishes activity of this system (as measured by reduced isolation induced distress vocalisations), could provisionally be regarded as a reasonable neurobiological vector for promoting autistic aloofness. For example, brain opioids are especially effective in reducing separation-induced distress vocalisations, and a child's self-imposed social isolation may arise in part, from overactivity of that system (Pankseep and Lensing, 1989).

A remarkable amount of congruence was noticed between the prominent symptoms of autistic individuals and animal treated with opiates. Moreover, the similarities between the symptoms are by no means restricted to social symptoms, but encompass the wide spectrum of behavioural and bodily changes that characterise autism, permitting both the emotional and cognitive changes to be subsumed by the same neurochemical influence (Pankseep and Lensing, 1989). The similarities noticed between autistics and the animals which were treated with opiates are as follows (Pankseep and Lensing, 1989):

1. Marked reduction in crying response to social isolation
2. Reduced desire/need for social contact
3. Decrease in sensitivity to pain
4. Diminished clinging behaviour
5. Characterised by an "insistence on sameness"
6. Substantial changes in social play
7. Delays in developmental milestones
8. Increased incidence of seizures
9. Increase in stereotyped behaviours
10. Characterised by motor activities/mannerisms
11. Abnormal vestibular functioning
12. Slower auditory evoke potentials
13. Major changes in eating behaviour
14. Changes in aggression, especially within dominance relations.

On the basis of the evidences like the above Pankseep and Lensing (1989), further hypothesised, that any psychopharmaceutical which promotes indices of distress, may be deemed a logical avenue of therapeutic influence (i.e. Potentiation of "social need" should potentiate the emission of desired social behaviours by autistic individuals). As a result they advocated the administration of the opiate receptor antagonist naltrexone for the symptomatic treatment of autistic disorders.

Opiate blocking agents such as naltrexone and naloxane have exhibited clear potential for increasing social tendencies in experimental animals. They promote the emission of contact seeking calls, they can increase specific pro-social gestures like friendly tail-wagging in dogs (Pankseep et al., 1980, 1985 and 1988). Several investigations have revealed the beneficial effects of Naltrexone in the treatment of autism and related disorders (Pankseep and Lensing, 1989). The important findings of those studies are:

- — Naltrexone induced reduction in the total self-injurious behaviour in the case of each child treated (Herman et al., 1987).
- — Naltrexone resulted in tranquillising effects such as significant reductions in restlessness and negative/uncooperative behaviour; Verbal production was also increased; high dose level resulted in strong reduction in stereotypes and significantly increased relatedness to others (Campbell et al., 1989).
- — In both children hyperactivity was rapidly and strikingly reduced when naltrexone was administered; social behaviour — eye contact, smiles, interactions — improved; self-injurious behaviour decrease and no side effects were noticed (Leboyer et al., 1988).

Pankseep and Lensing (1989) observed that naltrexone is most effective:

- — when given in low infrequent doses, and
- — when given in the presence of actively supportive and socially encouraging companion.

They strongly believe that there are two distinct therapeutic phases which follows naltrexone administration:

(1) During the acute phase, when opiate receptors are optimally blocked, there are major reductions of the active symptoms of autism such as stereotypes, hyperactivity,

self-injurious behaviours, and aggressiveness. (2) When opiate blocking should be waning over several hours there is, prominent enhancement of active pro-social behaviours such as vocalisations, face grazing, active touch and playfulness.

Shattock (1989) remarked that opioid excess theory may or may not be the solution to the riddle of autism but it does provide a convenient and logical explanation to link the many biochemical, emotional and psychological findings which have been reported separately over the years; it could point the way to appropriate, rational medical and behavioural interventions to reduce the negative consequences of autism without excess of side effects of other difficulties which are currently observed.

CHAPTER 4

Psycho-physiological Theories

Information processing deficit theories can be included under psycho-physiological theories. The basic theoretical assumptions, supportive empirical evidences, and the expected implications of information processing deficit theories are discussed below.

The hypothesis that the peculiar manner in which autistic children handle environmental stimuli is mainly due to physiological abnormalities in responsiveness and selective attention was one of the important theoretical issues in the past decades (Engeland, 1989). Anthony (1962) has observed three main theoretical explanations for autism in the work of his contemporaries — a derangement of sensory input, an interference with central co-ordinating and integrating mechanisms, a disorder of output. As per the opinion of Hermalin and O'Connor (1970), although this kind of categorisation is general and might correspond with a logically determined subdivision, the disorganisation of sensory input and central organisation can be considered as a basic model for autism. The basis for this theoretical point of view is Piaget's (1954) idea that in the autism of infancy there is an adualistic confusion between self and non-self. As summarised by Hermalin and O'Connor (1970), the autistic child has no sense of time and his sensory input structure lacks hierarchical organisation; he deals with the world in an adhoc fashion without reference to history, temporal series, or spatial organisation. In addition, he lacks language, which is essential to make it possible for a child to build a model of the world in the mind in a conceptual form (Bruner,

1957). According to them a confusion of sensory input combined with a lack of language could result in a state of autism.

Rimland (1964) strongly believed that autism results from a failure to integrate separate experiences. The stored material re-emerges unmodified, unlike the categorical store through which memorised material is normally processed. He designates this as "closed loop phenomena" suggesting that autism has a biogenic basis and is characterised by lack of integration of input and store.

According to Hermelin and O'Connor, the views of both Anthony and Rimland fall into the same kind of psychological theory of autism which presumes failure to develop "abstraction". This idea was originally used by Sheerer et al. (1945) to explain the idiot savant (learned fools). They suggested that certain children with symptoms resembling autism lack the capacity to think conceptually. Rimland has adapted this idea to account for certain aspects of autism like the tendency to arrange or order the external world, and the literalness or concreteness or verbal interpretation.

A number of research workers have suggested speculative physiological bases for the inability/disability among autistics to process the information. Ornitz (1970, 1971, 1974) postulated failure of adequate vestibular modulation of sensory input and output. Rimland (1964, 1968) suggested that malfunction of the reticular activating system (RAS) results in under-arousal to incoming stimuli with consequent inability to relate the new experiences to the ones already remembered. On the other hand Hutt and Hutt (1968) postulated that a chronically high level RAS activity causes blocking of sensory pathways.

Until recently, empirical research in the psychophysiology of childhood autism has produced rather conflicting results (Engeland, 1989). On the basis of a thorough review, James and Barry (1980) conclude that no characteristic feature of the functioning of the central nervous system can be unequivocally related to infantile autism. The single trend emerging from the data is that autistic children show responses that are different from those of normal children. The nature and direction of these differences can only be assumed.

Engeland and his colleagues engaged in physiological research about stimulus processing disorders and responsiveness to sensory stimuli in various subjects, including autistic children since about 1980. Engeland (1989) has given a thorough overview of developments in this research in his department and attempted to compare them with developments reflected in the literature. An attempt has been made below to give the essence of the same.

Most of the stimuli that reach us through our sensory organs are processed automatically and preconsciously with the aid of "preattentive mechanisms". Such automatic and continuous processing of the information takes place by comparing incoming stimuli with the "schemata" (substructures which are dynamically organised), neurological models or information on the context in which the organism is currently situated, and which is available to it at that moment (short-term memory).

When there is a discrepancy between the incoming stimulus and the available schema, but the stimulus is of greater importance to the individual in the present context, an orientation reaction occurs and the stimulus is passed onto a central channel of limited capacity. With the help of this central channel the short-term and long-term systems are scanned systematically, and may result in any one or both the results:

- The long-term memory proves to contain information which fits the incoming stimulus configuration, in which case this information is mobilised and made available to the short-term memory system (that means assimilation takes place).
- No information on the incoming stimulus is available in either system, in which case the organism is forced to accept the incoming stimulus information, to process it and to store it in the short-term memory system. New associations are then formed; schemata are constructed or renewed, and subsequently transported to the long-term memory system. In other words the organism accommodates to the newly incoming stimuli and builds a memory for them.

According to Ohman (1980), the occurance of an orientation reaction is conditional to learning. Without such a reaction the organism is unable to process information on structural changes in its environment and store it in its memory.

Repeated exposure to the same stimulus leads to the development of a neural model or "schema" of that stimulus, which enables the organism to find out whether the stimulus to which it is currently exposed is a familiar one or a novel one. If it is a familiar one, the orientation reaction towards that diminishes in strength and extinguishes on the other hand habituation to the stimulus occurs. The orientation process enables the organism to focus on environmental changes which may be of vital importance. Habituation ensures that the organism is not overwhelmed by stimuli; that it learns not to respond to stimuli which are irrelevant to the context. Thus orientation and habituation play an extremely important role in the adaptation of human beings to their environment.

Engeland and his coworkers compared 35 autistic children (mean age 8.9 years) with 39 normal children (mean age 8.9 years), 38 psychiatric patients (mean age 9.9 years) and 20 Down's syndrome (mean age 18.2 years) in electrodermal orientation reaction and event related potentials in response to auditory and visual stimuli. Eleven autistic children were severely mentally retarded; eleven others were mildly retarded, and the remaining showed IQs within the normal range.

On the basis of the above study the following conclusions were drawn by the investigators (Engeland, 1989):

- Autistic children suffer from a deficiency in processing novel and complex information. The information processing deficiency manifests itself in electrodermal reaction as well as in ERP.
- As far as the electrodermal parameters are concerned, autistic individuals seem to behave just like schizophrenic patients. Both the groups appear to be hypo-responsive to meaningless stimuli of high novelty value and do become normally responsive whenever subjective significance to those stimuli is added. This change in responsivity among autistic and schizophrenic patients does imply that there is no total loss of stimulus detection, filtering or orientation reaction capability per se. Motivational factors and effort seem to play a modulating role in stimulus responsiveness in these subjects.
- Deficits in stimulus detection as well as stimulus evaluation may account for most of the peculiarities in cognition and social behaviour of autistic children. Thus it seems

worthwhile to try to enhance orientation reaction in autistics which in turn might contribute to improvement in attentional and social behaviour among them.

In this connection some of the points raised by Shattock (1990) seems worth mentioning. First of all Shattock is of the opinion that in the past there had been an understandable tendency "not to concentrate" on perceptual problems. This could be because of the perceived necessity to differentiate autism from schizophrenia. Recently a number of people with autism, who have made dramatic progress, have been reporting sensory/perceptual irregularities in their earlier, more autistic phases (White, 1988 and Zoller, 1989). It is interesting to note there are certain similarities between those reports. The reported perceptual difficulties could be due to any of the following factors:

a. Faulty sensory input;
b. Faulty transmission of the input;
c. Faulty filtration/selection of data;
d. Difficulties in making comparison with "records" which may themselves be faulty.

Shattock (1990) suggests that it is possible to assume that all the four difficulties may exist to a greater or lesser extent in autistics. The process of filtration/selection of data is of particular importance to normal existence.

One possible consequence of defect in this process would be a deficit in the habituation process which can be noticed in event related potentials. As a result the individual is less effective in filtering out those stimuli which are significant from those which are not.

Shattock (1990) has made an attempt to apply this basic assumption to explain social and emotional behaviour among autistics. He hypothesises that if this filtration process is faulty for classical sensory inputs which will lead ultimately to cognitive difficulties it may be equally defective for emotional and social interpretations. Shattock attributes higher concentrations of peptides as responsible for defect in filtration/selection of data. Further he elaborates that the concentrations of peptides which will produce such effects that are termed as emotional, cognitive or social could well be much lower than those required to produce sensory aberrations. It is necessary to carefully evaluate the validity of such hypothesis in order to understand the true nature of autism.

CHAPTER 5

Psychological Theories

5.1 Introduction

The attempts to explore the psychological strengths and weaknesses of autistics and to explain the various autistic symptoms in terms of the observed deficits in the various psychological functions are too many compared to explanations in terms of biological, physiological or psychophysical defects. It is interesting to note that from global terms like cognition, information processing, memory, language disorders, etc. attempts have been made to make a finer analysis of the psychological functions that may be related to autistic syndrome. In fact compared to the other areas of work already discussed, verifying hypotheses related to psychological functions are much more complicated. Some of the reasons are general to any kind of psychological investigation. For example, conceptualisation of the psychological constructs. Different investigators might view the same construct from different angles and also some of them may be more comprehensive than the others. That means the construct validity may vary from study to study which make the comparison of the results unreliable. Similarly the problem of controlling factors within the population studied is also an important hazard to arrive at any definite conclusion regarding the psychological make up of the autistic individuals. Thirdly, autism is a complex syndrome with and multitude of symptoms, which can occur in many combinations and to any extent. Most probably this must be the major havoc in differentiating autism from other disabilities, mainly mental retardation, and aphasia, and to a considerable extent social-emotional problems of different kinds.

In fact the vast number of psychological investigations in the area of autism can be considered as a positive reaction of the investigators to the challenge posed by autism because of the above mentioned and many other problems. They really demand qualities like perseverance ingenuity, endurance, flexibility and originality. Attempts have been made fairly systematically and they are characterised by most of the qualities mentioned above. But in spite of such attempts they are not yet completely successful in explaining the enigma of autism, though some investigators are highly satisfied about their explanations, a lot of logical links are missing still. However a thorough review of the work done in this area should provide abundant information about the nature of autism.

Many investigators (Rutter, 1968; Hermelin, 1968; Mittler, 1968; Hermelin and O'Connor, 1970; Ricks and Wing, 1976; Hermelin, 1976; Demyer, 1976; Wing, 1976; Caplan and Walker, 1979; Rutter, 1983; Morgan, 1986; Clements, 1987; Baron-Cohen, 1988, 1990; Frith, 1989; Klin, 1989; Fein, 1989; Hobson, 1989; Gillberg, 1990; Klin, 1990, Roeck, 1990; Jordan, 1990) have given an extensive amount of investigations undertaken in different aspects of psychological development among autistics. As such there is no need to replicate the work. So an attempt has been made below only to report the important observations made and conclusions drawn by those authors. However, certain major theoretical assumptions are also elaborated and highlighted wherever necessary.

5.2 Language Impairment as a Major Defect

Rutter (1968) ascertained that infantile autism has nothing to do with schizophrenia and it is not primarily a disorder of social relationships. The presence of mental subnormality is not sufficient to account for autism and it seems unlikely that psychogenic or faulty conditioning mechanisms are primary causative factors, although they may play important role in the development of secondary handicaps. Further he has emphasised that of all the hypotheses the ones which consider language or coding problems as the primary defect among autistics appear most promising.

Hermelin (1966) also stressed that perhaps the most striking and most frequently occurring impairment in autistic children is their inability to handle language adequately, either as a mental tool or as a means of communication. However, she is cautious enough to highlight that it is not appropriate to consider one handicap as the primary one and all the others as secondary. She has also drawn attention to the fact that in the case of autistic child the functions are not simply underdeveloped, but distorted.

In her review Hermelin (1968) has quoted Luria's (1961) ideas about the nature of language impairment in the case of subnormal children. It is worth reproducing them here as they have their implications for the understanding of autism also.

Luria (1961) holds that the failure on the part of subnormal children to connect the verbal with the motor system is responsible for much of their cognitive deficits. In the opinion of Luria and his colleagues, the development of language turns simple differentiating/discriminating operations into reasoning processes, such as comparing. It is held that the verbal system in the severely subnormal children does not develop sufficiently to assume this orienting function. As a result words for such children remain only impelling excitatory signals, and there exists a dissociation between verbal and motor systems. Stimulus response connections which consequently become established without verbal associations tend to remain unstable and specific. In addition, they may depend on constant reinforcement, and disintegrate at a slight change in the manner of presenting the signals.

The real riddle starts here. If lack of abstraction among subnormal children as well as autistics are due to language impairment, what is the difference between autistics and subnormals ? Can we attribute the inability to abstract among autistics to subnormality in intelligence ? Mittler (1968) reported that intelligence test results among autistics, although by no means normally distributed around the mean do extend well above the subnormal range. The number of children who are just below average or even average in intelligence vary from 30% (Rutter, 1966) to 47% (Pollock, 1960). On an average at least 40% of the autistics are expected to have normal language development. As observed by Rutter (cited in Hermelin, 1968) a large proportion of autistic children do not speak at all; but even the child who does speak might still fail to develop normal language, though his actual vocabulary need not necessarily be limited.

Rutter's observation poses two questions. When he states that some autistics have sufficient vocabulary, does it cover not only simple and concrete concepts (merely labels) but also complex and abstract concepts ? If vocabulary in this context includes only labelling, that may not really help in abstract thinking. Secondly, if the development of language among autistics is not considered as normal in spite of sufficient vocabulary, in what way is it different ?

Various attempts have been made to answer this question either by comparing autistics with mentally retarded or normal or dysphasic controls. The dimensions of comparison are varied across different studies in this direction. The experimental studies by Hermelin and O'Connor (1970) clearly indicated that autistic youngsters markedly differed from normal or retarded children in many ways. The autistic child had immediate auditory rote memories which were better than those of subnormals and as good as, or better than, those of normal children of similar mental age. However, the recall capacity of the control groups improved significantly when syntactical and meaningfully related material was presented. But there was no such difference in the case of autistics. There was little difference in recall of sense or nonsense in the autistic group. On the other hand, the autistic children showed stronger recency effects than the other groups.

The experiments by Hermelin and O'Conner (1970) further revealed that the autistic children did not vary in the amount of responsiveness according to the nature of the stimuli, whether sounds or words. While phonological stress on words had the same facilitating effect on recall as it had for other children, the difference between recall efficiency of words arranged into sentences and randomly arranged word sequences was far less marked in the autistic than in the normal and subnormal children.

Rutter (1983) thinks that out of the two questions — "what cognitive deficits may be associated with autism ?" and "what cognitive deficits must be present for autism to develop ?", the latter is more appropriate. In order to answer the acceptable question two research strategies can be adopted. The first strategy involves the study of autistic children of normal non-verbal intelligence in whom autism occurs in a "pure' form, and is not associated with mental retardation or other handicaps.

Rutter (1983) has pointed out that the other approach that was employed by some authors is to draw parallels between autism and developmental dysphasia and to suggest that some form of language deficit might be primary to autism. He remarks that the premise behind this approach is to suggest that autism might be a consequence of a defect in the understanding of language and in the cognitive processes that deal with language and language-related functions and not certainly to imply that autism could be a consequence of speech abnormalities. The important question to be answered is what cognitive defects are responsible for the language abnormalities and behavioural characteristics of autistics?

Rutter (1983) recommends that this question can be tackled by comparing autistics with dysphasics of comparable level of IQ and language development. He has reported the results of studies undertaken by him and Bartak, which are summarised below.

Firstly, it was clear that the two groups differed considerably more in their social and behavioural characteristics than some of the earlier clinical descriptions had suggested (Bartak et al., 1975). There is sufficient evidence to conclude that a receptive language disorder is not sufficient to account for the autistic syndrome.

Secondly, there were some important cognitive and language features on which the autistic children were not disadvantaged compared with the 'dysphasic' children. The groups did not differ in non-verbal reasoning skills or in syntactic language skills, and the autistic children were actually less impaired on measures of articulation (Boucher, 1976; Cantwell et al., 1978). The findings indicate that it is most unlikely that the basis of autism lies in any general deficit in visuo-spatial or perceptual cognition, articulation or the grammatical aspects of language. Similar conclusions were drawn on the basis of the findings from other studies (DeMyer et al., 1981).

Thirdly, there were a number of features on which the autistic children were significantly more handicapped (Bartak et al., 1975; Cantwell et al., 1978). They are as follows:

- The language disorder of the autistic children was both more severe and more persistent;
- The dysphasic children, unlike the autistic group, were not impaired in the so-called 'inner language' functions, as revealed through cognitive measures that required 'verbal-type' skills in thought processes;
- Study of imaginative play and the use and understanding of gesture indicated that the language deficit in autism is far broader than that in 'dysphasia';
- With reference to the use of speech for social communication, unlike 'dysphasic' children, few autistic children were able to hold a proper conversation with a reciprocal and responsive to and fro interchange; moreover, this deficit remained even after they had gained clearly adequate language skills for the purpose;
- Autistic children differed in showing various abnormal features of language, especially inappropriate echoing of what they themselves had just said and other forms of stereotyped and a typical language usage.

On the basis of the above observations Rutter (1983) concludes that autism is associated with both language abnormalities and a cognitive deficit that was more severe, more widespread and somewhat different in pattern from that found in developmental 'dysphasia'. The cognitive abnormalities were indeed of a kind linked with language, but they extended well beyond spoken language; moreover, it appeared to be language deviance as much as language delay that was characteristic of autism.

Rutter (1983) emphasised two language characteristics of autism. The first one is the autistic child's relative failure to use language for social communication; autistic individuals may learn to talk fluently and, indeed, some autistic adults develop considerable language fluency and talk almost excessively. But still they tend to bombard their conversational partners with rather stereotyped statements and questions rather than converse in the reciprocal-responsive fashion that is typical of the language interchanges of even very young normal children. The second observation is that long after autistic individuals gain fluent language and cease to show the gross cognitive deficits that characterised them when younger, they remain obviously abnormal in their social interactions (Rutter, 1970). He recommended that there is a need to focus research more explicitly on the characteristics of autistic children's social impairments and on the possible cognitive deficits that might underlie them.

5.3 Social and Pragmatic Deficits in Autism

Baron-Cohen (1988) has given an extensive review of the theoretical assumptions and also the results of many studies relating to the social and pragmatic deficits among autistics. Bates (1976) has defined pragmatics as the use of speech and gesture in a communicative way, appropriate to the social context. This implies that pragmatic skills are part of the social skills, as such, whatever underlies the deficit in social skills is also likely to underlie the deficit in pragmatic skills.

Wing and Gould (1979) have distinguished social impairment into three types — social aloofness, passive interaction, and active-but-odd interaction. The latter category suggests social behaviour that is repetitive, idiosyncratic preoccupation, showing no interest in the other person's needs. They observed that only 70% of their autistic subjects showed aloofness whereas the remaining 30% fell into the other categories of social impairment.

Wing (1978) reported that the full, classic picture of aloofness and detachment seems much more marked in the younger autistic child, of less than 5 years old. Hopkins and Lord (1981) consider the three categories of social impairment identified by Wing and Gould are useful descriptions for rating the autistic children. They found that the category which any autistic child falls into differs according to his/her age, sex, familiarity, and diagnosis of the playmate. They concluded that an autistic child's social impairment thus takes different forms according to who they are with, but it nevertheless persists. The impairment also changes developmentally. Lord (1984) indicated a progression from "aloof" to "passive" in social responsiveness, and from "aloof" to "passive" to "odd" in rate of initiation of interaction.

On the basis of a thorough review of studies relating to social behaviour and social understanding of autistic children Baron-Cohen (1988) summarised the findings as follows:

- Studies on autistic children's social behaviour document the chronic nature of the social deficit, and suggest that although it may change its form both developmentally and across situations, an inability to participate in two-way reciprocal social interaction persists throughout the lives of autistic people.
- The studies of autistic children's social understanding have shown a number of unimpaired areas, such as face recognition, mirror self-recognition (Flannery, 1976; Neuman and Hill, 1978; Ferrari and Mathews, 1983; Spiker and Ricks, 1984; Dawson and McKissick, 1984; Baron-Cohen, 1985) and perceptual role-taking (Hobson, 1984; Baron-Cohen, 1985). But severe impairments have been found in intermodal matching of emotional expressions, in conceptual role-taking (Baron-Cohen, Leslie and Frith, 1985), specifically in attributing different beliefs to others, and in imitation of abstract gestures (Curcio, 1978; Hammes and Langdell, 1981).

Finally, he recommends that an important task for psychological theories in this area is to explain why autistic children's social understanding assumes particularly uneven profile.

Cunningham (1968) has classified the autistic child's speech as "egocentric" and "socialised", and found more egocentric remarks in autistic children's speech than in matched controls. Egocentric speech reflected echolalia, self-repetition, thinking aloud, and apparently purposeless remarks. Cunningham has discussed the excessive egocentric speech in terms of Piaget's (1932) theory of young normal children's egocentricism, and concluded that autism may represent an immaturity of development. Cunningham (1968) has expressed his ideas as follows:

- As Piaget (1932) points out, the exchange of information requires the speaker to place himself at the point of view of his hearer. This the psychotic (autistic) child is unable to do. He shows a lack of empathy or ability to apprehend his hearer's state of mind and therefore falls back on non-communicative or demanding speech.

Baron-Cohen (1988) has reviewed studies relating to pragmatic defects among autistics. He thinks that the term pragmatics was not used in most of the earlier studies. However, they describe certain defects which will fall in the category of pragmatic difficulties. The important observations made by him on the findings of those studies are as follows:

- Autistic children frequently failed to shift out of the hearer role to become a speaker (Baltaxe, 1977); (she has quoted one of her autistic subjects: "Well, I asked my parents. I told my parents I'd be good at home, but I feel you're too old to be at home, we feel you should be away").
- Baltaxe also found that autistic subjects violated "conversational postulates" of acceptability and politeness (Bates, 1976), not because they intended to be rude, but simply because they did not understand the social rules governing what is acceptable in conversation.
- The autistic adolescents tended not to "foreground and background" their utterances; that is, their choice of words did not allow the listener to differentiate between old and new information (Baltaxe, 1977).
- Baltaxe and Simmons (1977) studied the bedtime soliloquies of an autistic girl and found that the girl tended to make her speech a monologue, whereas normal children often act out of two-way conversation (Weir, 1962).
- Bernard-Opitz (1982) found that an autistic child's language did vary as a function of the interlocutor (i.e. whether it was mother, stranger, or clinician), showing some social sensitivity, while nevertheless revealing pragmatic deficits, such as perseveration on a topic.
- Hurtling, Ensrud, and Tomblin (1982) manipulated another variable, namely, listener-response to questions. They found that more conversational breakdowns (discontinuations) occurred if the listener did not ask a question back to the child, suggesting that the autistic children were unable to maintain the conversation by themselves. In addition, the autistic children appeared to use questions as their main device to initiate and continue conversation, but tended to ask questions to which they already knew the answers. They appear not to understand the function of questions as requests for information.

- Whetherby (1986) asserts that autistic children are communicative, as they use language in an intentional way towards another person to achieve environmental or social ends (Whetherby, 1986; Prizant, 1983 & 1984). He takes support from the findings of the studies by Prizant and Duchan (1981) and Prizant and Rydell (1984) that autistic children's echolalia functions as expressions of intentions to request, protest, affirm, etc.

Baron-Cohen (1988) reacts to the justification of Wetherby — that there is no dispute that autistic children can use language intentionally by raising a question whether this evidence is sufficient to conclude that they are communicative? He quotes Speech Act Theory (Austin, 1962; Searle, 1965) which defines communication as comprising "complex intentions" — that is, the speaker's intention to affect the listener's intentions and beliefs. Thus speaker's intentions represent only one side of communication.

CHAPTER 6

Explanations to Social and Pragmatic Deficits among Autistics

The social and pragmatic deficits that are quite obvious among autistics are attributed to cognitive and non-cognitive aspects of development among them. The important postulates of those theories are discussed below.

6.1 Cognitive Theories

The cognitive theories which are concerned with the characteristic features among autistics are mainly of two types. One set of theories are quite comprehensive and attempt to explain most of the salient features of autistics. Piaget's Two-Factor Theory, as proposed by Morgan (1986), is one such theory. On the other hand some theories mainly restrict themselves to social and pragmatic deficits among autistics. The Metarepresentation Theory (Baron-Cohen, 1988; Frith, 1989) falls under this category. An attempt has been made here to review the important ideas, recommendations and implications of those theories.

6.1.1 Piaget's Two-Factor Theory and Autistic Syndrome

As an introduction to his discussion on the compatibility between Piaget's Two-Factor Theory and Autism, Morgan (1986), has considered the following cognitive dysfunctions as central to autism.

— defect in sensorimotor integration (Ornitz, 1976, 1979);

— an inability to relate present to past experience (Rimland, 1964);

— a pervasive language disorder (Churchill, 1978);
— an impairment in using symbols (Ricks and Wing, 1975);
— an inability to interpret social and emotional cues (Rutter, 1983).

Morgan is of the opinion that the above conceptions do not have a common theoretical base. He thinks it might be useful to analyse the features of autism within the framework of Piaget's cognitive model. The justification he has given for applying Piaget's theory of cognitive development to explain autistics syndrome are:

— it is possible to trace more precisely the course of aberrations in the autistic child's cognitive development;
— Piaget's detailed account of cognitive development during infancy seems particularly applicable to infantile autism; such an analysis may also help to assess and appreciate the complexities of normal intellectual development as certain cognitive functions appear to be impaired in autistic children;
— further, a look at autism from this perspective should stress the reciprocal relationship between cognitive development and affective-social development;
— finally, a Piagetian analysis of autism would serve as a preliminary test of generality of the theory and its scope to explain the deviations and inconsistencies that distinguish the autistic child from the normal child and the non-autistic mentally retarded child.

Morgan has reviewed the various studies (Thatcher, 1977; Wing et al., 1977; Curcio, 1978; Rosenthal, Massie, and Wulf, 1980; Hammes and Langdell, 1981; Sigman and Ungerer, 1984) which have attempted to determine whether autistic children show deficits in functioning at Piaget's sensorimotor level. On the basis of the findings of those studies Morgan has inferred that it seems reasonable to assume that autism involves a cognitive arrest in some functions at the sensorimotor level rather than a regression of functions to this stage.

On the basis of the observations made in certain studies, Morgan (1986), concluded that in autism the cognitive dysfunctions emerge at a very early stage of cognitive development and persist thereafter (Wing et al., 1977; Rosenthal et al., 1980; Hammes and Langdell, 1981; Sigman and Ungerer, 1984).

The important hypothesis that emerges from the observations made in the studies on cognitive development of autistic children is the one proposed by Sigman and Ungerer (1984). Their hypothesis is "Autism involves deficits in certain object concepts and not in others. Representational thought may be revealed in two different systems. One system involves the capacity to recall information, while the other involves the capacity to form and manipulate symbols. In normal and retarded children, these two systems develop together, whereas in autistic children the two systems diverge, with the latter being arrested." In fact Caplan and Walker (1979) firmly believed that autistic children cannot progress from static symbolic representation to transformational representation. The explanation they have given for such an inability is their deficiency in symbolic imagery which in turn leads to severe difficulty in focusing on or relating several dimensions simultaneously.

The conclusion drawn by Caplan and Walker (1979) and also the hypotheses proposed by Sigman and Ungerer (1984), thus supports the possibility of applying Piaget's Two-Factor Theory to explain autistic syndromes. According to Piaget (1964 & 1968), the operative aspect of cognition refers to actions whose results are some transformation or change of reality; the figurative aspect refers to actions by which the child reproduces or represents a "copy" of reality; concentration, then, is upon the state of reality rather than transformations.

Morgan (1986) raises an important question concerning how far Piaget's theory explains the atypical, seemingly paradoxical, cognitive development of autistic individuals. He has attempted himself to answer this question in the following way. The paradoxical cognitive profile of the autistic children not only differs from the consistent pattern of most retarded children but also appears to be inconsistent with generalised cognitive arrest at the sensorimotor level. In addition, the developmental sequence appears to depart from what Piaget calls "semiotic function", which comprises the following modes in order of developmental complexity — deferred imitation, symbolic play, drawing or graphic representation, mental imagery or imagination, and spoken and written language (Cowan, 1976). Morgan has made the paradox clear with an example: Is it possible that an autistic child never develops symbolic play but achieves higher levels of the semiotic function such as spoken language?

Morgan (1986) has continued his analysis with the statement that these apparent exceptions to the sequence of semiotic function exhibited by autistic children are difficult to explain with the similar sequence hypothesis if cognitive development is strictly considered unidimensional. He has proposed that they might be explained, through Piaget's two-factor theory of symbolic meaning (Cowan, 1978), which differentiates representation (the figurative aspect of symbols) from conceptualisation (the operative aspect of symbols). Through representation, the individual encodes, stores, and retrieves accurate images of specific events. Figurative schemes, therefore, correspond to the configuration of the events represented and primarily accommodative as they are formed to repeat aspects of a particular event. In contrast, conceptualisation involves the operative aspect of symbols. A specific representational image cannot assume meaning until it is incorporated into a general conceptual structure or scheme that, as distinguished from figurative schemes, is primarily assimilative and operative. In normal cognitive development, meaningful symbols are formed as a product of interaction between accommodation and assimilation to achieve dynamic equilibrium.

The highlights of the implications of Piaget's two-factor theory to explain the salient features of autism (Morgan, 1986) are as follows:

- The autistic child's seemingly bizarre motor behaviour and lack of symbolic play may be explained by an arrest of certain operative functions at the sensorimotor level. The posturing and flapping of hands are not so unusual if seen as primary circular reactions.
- The repetitive and stereotypic manipulation of objects, including toys, is in many respects comparable to secondary circular reactions; the autistic child seems to be trying to assimilate objects by forcing them into some sensorimotor scheme.
- The preservation of primitive responses and the failure to develop symbolic play in autism, cannot be explained just from mental age as assessed by traditional psychometric

measures as the studies by Wing et al. (1977), Riguet et al. (1981), and Sigman and Ungerer (1984) clearly showed that more deficits in symbolic play occur in autistic than retarded children of comparable mental ages.

— The inconsistency between mental age or IQ and the development of flexible symbolic functioning in autistic children might be explained by the so-called splinter skills that give spuriously high estimates of their conceptual functioning. An examination of these skills reveals a strong figurative component with minimal operative functioning.

— The spatial and perceptual-motor skills are usually tested on fitting and assembly tasks that require rote manipulation or reproduction of objects rather than flexible handling of symbols.

— The graphic skills found in some autistic individuals usually represent rote reproduction of environmental configurations rather than reflect any creative expression.

— The memory skills demonstrated on such tests as digit span seem rote replications of auditory stimuli with little utilisation of meaning.

— On tests that require symbolic fluidity they usually perform quite poorly. Their isolated performance peaks on traditional IQ measures, thus, appear to reflect figurative rather operative functioning.

— Speech development in many autistic children also presents a paradox that is difficult to resolve without resort to the two-factor theory. Spoken and written language represents the highest level of the semiotic function. The crucial distinction for autism, is between speech and language. Many autistic children appear to learn to speak but rarely go beyond the figurative aspects of speech to the operative characteristics of language. Although they may speak with good articulation, they show deficits in prosodic and semantic features of language as well as an inability to switch linguistic codes (Baltaxe and Simmons, 1975; Boucher, 1976). They also exhibit deficits in concept formation (Noach, 1974) and an overwhelming dependence on imitation in linguistic coding (Shapiro and Kapit, 1978) Further, it was noticed that majority of autistic children fail to develop true spontaneous speech, even with intensive behavioural training (Lovaas,

1977; Carr, 1979; Prior, 1979). These features of autistic speech suggest that the figurative aspects appear, in most cases, to be no higher than the lowest level of the semiotic function, that is, deferred imitation.

— The seemingly precocious reading skill, or hyperplexia, exhibited by some autistic children also appears to be applied in a figurative sense (Cobrink, 1974; Whitehouse and Harris, 1984). Such children show an isolated facility for decoding written material without comprehension of its meaning. This ability, which far exceeds expectations based on the child's general intelligence, is associated with unusually good visual and auditory memory and stored vocabulary within the context of poor expressive and receptive language (Whitehouse and Harris, 1984).

— The autistic child who speaks or reads but fails to engage in symbolic play probably does not speak or read in any operative, conceptual way. Thus it is possible to propose that autistic children, in their cognitive development, do adhere to the similar sequence hypothesis in a strict operative, conceptual sense, and many fail to progress beyond the sensorimotor level in operative skills. Those who do develop the flexible use of symbols and language will have passed through a conceptual sequence which is not different from that of normal or retarded individuals. Research on early predictors of long-term adjustment in autistic individuals supports this conclusion; the early skills are highly correlated with later adjustment, such as communicative speech and appropriate play behaviour, reflect some attainment of operative functioning (Brown, 1960; Lotter, 1978).

— Although the cognitive anomalies in autism might be explained on the basis of a substantial discrepancy between figurative and operative functions, it seems quite difficult to apply the same understanding to explain the most salient and disturbing feature of autistic children, that is, the failure to achieve normal social attachments and develop normal social interactions. Rutter (1983) has clearly stated that the autistic child's social anomalies stem from some special cognitive defect in dealing with social and emotional clues — a defect not found in the child with typical retardation. A basic question, then, is whether such a defect can be explained in terms of concepts already available in cognitive-developmental theory.

— Two early landmarks in normal cognitive development that may be relevant to the affective and social deficits of autistic children are the object concept and symbolic play. Piaget (1953, 1955) gave substantial importance to the object concept, considering it the earliest expression of processes that provide the substrate for later development of reasoning, logical thinking, and language. In normal children, attachment appears to be related to level of development of object permanence (Lester et al., 1974). The study by Hammes and Langdell (1981) has demonstrated that autistic children were much more inflexible and "stimulus-bound" than retarded children in manipulating internalized images both across modalities and across time. The findings suggest that autistic children may not achieve a stable concept of object constancy. This inability to anticipate states of objects may extend to people, who represent perhaps the most unpredictable of objects in the child's world. The autistic child forms attachments and clings to predictable objects but resists those (including people) that are least predictable.

— A defect in object constancy, then, might undermine the formation of stable social attachments and interfere with development of more advanced cognitive activities, such as symbolic play, that are necessary for normal social development. Sigman and Ungerer (1984) found that attachment and symbolic play were positively correlated in autistic children; that is, the autistic child who showed more attachment behaviours was also capable of a higher level of symbolic play.

After such a thorough analysis of the essential features of autism within the framework of Piagetian two-factor theory, it is highly appropriate that Morgan (1986) has suggested a series of research questions. The important questions are as follows:

- Does autism represent an exception to the similar sequence hypothesis that cannot be explained by Piaget's Two-Factor Theory?
- Do autistic individuals reveal clear and consistent differences in performance on tasks measuring figurative func-

tions versus those measuring operative functions?

- Do they demonstrate a greater discrepancy between figurative and operative functions than normal persons and those with cognitive impairments such as mental retardation and developmental aphasia?
- Do traditional tests with strong figurative components overestimate adaptive cognitive functioning in the Piagetian sense?
- Which type of measure better predicts adaptation to the real world and long-term adjustment?
- On Piagetian tasks do we find as much variability in cognitive functioning in a group of autistic individuals as we find on psychometric tests?
- Do some autistic individuals remain primarily at the sensorimotor level in operative functioning while others perform at the preoperational or concrete operational or higher level?

Morgan (1986) has concluded that in order to answer these questions it is essential to develop more refined Piagetian assessment techniques which assess such cognitive phenomena as object constancy, symbolic play, and conservation in children with disorders such as autism.

Piaget's Two Factor Theory as discussed by Morgan (1986) seems to be adequate to explain most of the crucial aspects relating to Deviance in Development of Social Relationships, Abnormalities in Communication, as well as Restricted, Repetitive and Stereotyped Patterns of Behaviour among autistic individuals. However it does not make any attempt to explain another important characteristic feature of autism — Sensory Deviation. That means it cannot answer questions like the following:

1. Why do autistics fail to recognise things seen?
2. Why do they use peripheral vision?
3. What is the reason for visual avoidance among autistics?
4. Why there is apparent non-reaction to noise among them?
5. Why do autisitics fail to react to a loud noise behind but how can they respond to rustle of a thin paper?
6. What makes them to avoid loud noises or speech?
7. Why do autistics exhibit indifference to pain/cold, inability to localise a sensation, unusual tastes or interests in unusual smells?

8. Why do they try to identify objects through licking, tapping, etc. rather than through sight or hearing?

The next important question which is difficult to be explained by Piaget's Two-Factor Theory (Morgan, 1986), is how can different sensory deviations affect operative aspect only leaving figurative aspect of cognitive development intact? Or else, are autistics with normal figurative development relatively free from deviation at least in some of the sensory functions, mainly visual and auditory?

It seems there is no answer in Morgan's (1986) postulates with reference to autism, even to the following questions:

— Is autism a permanent condition like mental retardation implying that it cannot be cured or controlled?
— There are certain evidences where in autistics are reported to have recovered at least partially or to considerable extent, if not totally. If they recover during later childhood/adolescence adulthood, what happens to their cognitive development? Do they exhibit operative skills after recovery?
— Is there any relationship between level of cognitive development with reference to operative thinking during childhood and also possibility of recovering from autism in the later stages of development? What skills/aspects of development remain deficient even after considerable "recovery"?
— Is significant discrepancy between figurative and operative aspects of cognitive development form a unique distinguishing feature of autism?

In addition to the above lacuna the Piagetian Two-Factor Theory (Morgan, 1986) as an explanation to autistic syndrome does not reveal any signs of encompassing possible emotional problems/physical health problems among autistic individuals. It does not try to establish any causal relationship between possible physiological disorders and delay/deficit in operative aspect of cognitive development.

In spite of its limitations Piagetian Two-Factor Theory (Morgan, 1986) has important implications for education of autistic children. Some of them are as follows:

1. assessment of cognitive development can be a better indicator of autistic child's academic performance;

2. instructional objectives can be set more realistically with the help of knowledge of level and nature of cognitive development;
3. instructional methods should utilise figurative capabilities effectively in order to develop various daily living and academic skills;
4. deliberate attempts should be made to foster operative skills among autistics;
5. as autistics are different from mentally retarded children in their cognitive development with the consequent differences in cognitive styles and preferences they should be taught in special classes meant for autistic children rather than club them with mentally retarded children;
6. as there is much heterogeneity among autistics individualised educational programmes are desirable wherever necessary;
7. extent of cognitive development with respect to figurative and operative skills separately and the discrepancy between these two types of skills may form criteria for grouping autistics among themselves, or with normal children or with specific learning disabled ones.

6.1.2 Meta-Representation Theory

In fact the well known concepts like "theory of mind" (Wimmer and Perner, 1983), "second order representations" (Dennet, 1978; Johnson-Laird, 1983) or "meta-representations" (Leslie, 1987; Pylyshyn, 1978), fit very well into the concepts of Guilford and Hoepfner (1966) namely "behavioural information" and "convergent thinking". Theory of mind, implies the ability to attribute mental states with content to others and meta-representations indicate our beliefs about other people's mental states. Convergent thinking means generation of information from given information, wherein the emphasis is on achieving unique or conventionally accepted best outcomes. It is likely that the given behavioural information (cue) fully determines the response to arrive at "implications". According to Guilford and Hoepfner (1966) implications refer to extrapolations of information, in the form of expectancies, predictions, known or suspected antecedents, concomitants, or consequences. Thus the theoretical assumption that in autism the capacity for meta-representations is impaired (Baron-Cohen, 1988) indirectly suggests that autistics have serious difficulty in dealing with "behavioural information" through the application of "convergent thinking" to arrive at "implications". As convergent thinking with reference to behavioural information is deficit consequently divergent thinking and evaluative thinking also will be deficient.

Baron-Cohen (1988) has attempted to summarise meta-representation theory in the form of five axioms which are indicated below.

1. Autism is caused by central cognitive deficits.
2. One such deficit is in the capacity for meta-representation.

3a. A meta-representational capacity is required in social skills which involve attributing mental states such as beliefs and desires to others (i.e. using a "theory of mind"). Such social skills will therefore be impaired in autism.

3b. Social skills which do not require a meta-representational capacity may be unimpaired in autism.

4. A meta-representational capacity is required in symbolic skills (e.g. pretend play).
5. Almost all pragmatic skills require a theory of mind (which itself requires a meta-representational capacity). These will therefore also be impaired in autism.

The meta-representation theory tries to explain social and pragmatic deficits unidirectionally. It does not emphasise the impact of deficient social and pragmatic skills in turn on development of theory of mind. Is not social and pragmatic skills on one hand and development of theory of mind on the other hand reciprocal in nature? Normal persons develop theory of mind through dynamic interaction with other individuals. So why can't we reason out that the "aloofness" and "passiveness" on the part of autistics impair meta-representational skills among them?

The above analysis reveal that the relationship between meta-representational skills and socio-pragmatic skills is not linear in nature, but definitely imply a circular relationship. Because of this kind of relationship it is difficult to understand which is more basic — whether deficiency in meta-representational skills or in socio-pragmatic skills? In fact, the meta-representation theory assumes the former as the most basic deficit, but does not attempt to explain why autistics have such a deficiency? This is the important limitation of this theory.

Any how by comparing the axioms of meta-representation theory with the three dimensional model of intellect proposed by Guilford, it can be understood that autistics have difficulty not only in dealing with behavioural information but also with semantics (pragmatics). This is because of the intricate relationship between the two types of contents namely semantics and behaviours. It follows from this that execution of operations in these areas to arrive at higher order products are significantly impaired among autistics.

6.2 Affective Theory

Hobson (cited in Baron-Cohen, 1986) strongly believes that — "On a number of levels, autism should be counted as a disorder of affective and social relations — and irreducibly so". He summarised his theory in terms of four major axioms which are reproduced below.

1. Autistic children lack the constitutional components of action and reaction which are necessary for the development of reciprocal personal relations with other people, relations which involve feelings.
2. Such personal relations are necessary for 'constitution of an own and common world' with others.
3. Autistic children's lack of participation in inner subjective social experience has two results which are especially important, namely (a) a relative failure to recognize other people as people with their own feelings/thoughts, wishes, intentions, and so on, and (b) a severe impairment in the capacity to abstract and feel and think symbolically.
4. The greater part of autistic children's cognitive and language disability may be seen to reflect either lower-order deficits that have a specially intimate relationship with affective and social development, and/or impairments in the social-dependent capacity to symbolize.

It is interesting to note that meta-representation theory tries to explain social and pragmatic deficits in terms of impaired meta-representational skills, whereas affective theory attributes impairment in meta-representational skills to lack of reciprocal relationship with others. Both the theories sound to be logical, mainly because there exists reciprocal relationship between cognitive skills and social skills. The limitations of these two theories are that they attempt to explain a one-way relationship but not the two-way one. The evidence for determining whether socio-emotional deficits lead to meta-representational deficiencies or vice versa in the case of autistics is not sufficient.

The theories, in general, emphasise the co-existing nature of cognitive and affective deficits among autistic individuals. The Piagetrian Two-Factor Theory (Morgan, 1986) as well the meta-representational theory (Baron-Cohen, 1988) suggest that there is unidimensional development of cognitive skills in the case of autistics rather than the expected two-dimensional development. According to Two-Factor Theory Figurative aspect and as per Meta-representational theory "Primary Representations" are quite adequate whereas Operative Functions and "Second Order Representations" are impaired respectively in autistics. The affective theory stresses the lack of development of interpersonal relationship among autistics with other individuals. Hobson (cited in Baron-Cohen, 1988) postulates that this is a constitutionally determined disability. He does not consider possibility of exogenous factors as also causes for impaired interpersonal relations in the case of autistic individuals.

6.3 Inner Language Among Autistics

While discussing about the significance of a language deficit hypothesis among autistics Rutter (1983), has remarked that "this hypothesis was tenable, but it proved to be potentially misleading in that it necessarily invoked concepts of "inner language" and of the thought processes underlying language. This constituted a problem because, although obviously there are such thought processes, there is no very straight forward way of deciding which thought processes are or are not language related". From the second part of the statement it is clear that thought he agrees with the concept of "inner language", he is doubtful about the relevance of different psycholinguistic processes which are thought to underlie language skills. A similar opinion is expressed by Mittler and Ward (1970) based on the findings of their study regarding the validity of ITPA in tapping specific psycholinguistic skills. They have concluded that a single general factor accounts for about 45% of the variance. This implies that there exists a high correlation between different aspects of language, such as development of concepts, attaining various syntax patterns, gaining meaning from meaningful pictures, organisation and communication of the ideas in a logical sequence. In fact the term "inner language" becomes an umbrella term which encompasses all these aspects of language.

Myklebust (1960) has pointed out that the three steps in the acquisition of language are the development of inner language or meaningfulness, auditory receptive language, and auditory expressive language.

According to Goldstein (1948), inner language is that language we use to communicate with ourselves, whereas Johnson and Myklebust (1967) conceives it as the language we use to think. Wallace and Kauffman (1973) have suggested that "inner language is dependent upon the child's ability to: (i) establish imagery for sounds, words, concepts, etc. (ii) use the complex maze of skills needed in the logical thinking process".

Sheridan (1969) has suggested that the beginnings of inner language can be seen in the normal child of around 12 months in age, at the same time he is beginning to understand a few words in context. At this stage he shows that he understands the use of real everyday objects by applying them to himself, for example brushing his own hair with a brush. By 18 months he uses the objects appropriately in relation to other people or pets and, by 2 years he is able to use correctly miniature objects such as a doll's tea set. The further development of inner language can be seen as play becomes more and more complex. It reveals the level at which the child is able to symbolise and abstract and the extent to which he can understand new events by matching them against his coded store of past experiences, using this comprehension as a basis of for further action. In older children and adults this sort of inner language is no longer revealed in play, but may be judged on conversation, observations of behaviour and knowledge of the interests of the persons.

Ricks and Wing (1976), consider that development of inner language is very poor among autistic children, and such a poverty forms an important feature among them. They give some justification for this hypothesis, on the basis of their clinical experience. Their important observations are:

— Most young autistic children handle toys and other objects as if they are seeking sensory stimuli; they do not use them for their proper purpose or for imaginative play.
— They may be able to do jig-saw and assemble constructional toys, as long as they require only visuo-spatial or mechanical skills and not imaginative understanding.
— Those who read from choice tend to use this skill to acquire facts about subjects who are interesting to them; however, works of fiction have little appeal, probably because a rich inner life, dependent upon inner language, is necessary for their enjoyment.
— Even the brighter autistic adolescents do not show signs of appropriate planning for the future and lack of interest in the realities of adult life; this type of foresight depends upon the existence of inner language which can be used for thinking and planning.

Though the above observations appear to be valid, it is difficult to accept their generalizability unless systematic attempts are made to explore the inner language among autistic children and adolescents.

Ramaa and Mittler (1991) conducted a study on "verbal autistics" with the objective of developing an insight into the "inner language" among them. The term "verbal autistics" refers to those autistic students who were quite capable of using spoken language in day-to-day living, as judged by their teachers. Thus 25 autistics students were selected from 5 schools for such students in United Kingdom. The number of subjects so selected varied from school to school. The age of those subjects ranged from 6 years 6 months to 18 years and 11 months. There were 6 females and 19 males altogether in the study.

In the study by Ramaa and Mittler (1991), inner language among autistics was treated as represented by Vocabulary Development (BPVS — British Picture Vocabulary Scale, Dunn et al., 1982); Basic Concepts (BTBC — Boehm's Test of Basic Concepts, Boehm, 1969); Sentence Comprehension (SCT — entence Comprehension Test, Mittler et al., Wheldall, Mittler and Hobsbaum, 1987); and Ability to Arrange Pictures in Logical Sequence (PRT — Picture Arrangement Test, subtest of WISC, Wechsler, 1949). It was attempted to make a detailed analysis of the responses of autistics to the items of these tests and also to find out the extent to which their performance on BPVS is related to their performance on other tests. Only about the correlational aspect of the study is discussed below. Coefficients of correlation between Vocabulary Age/Raw Scores on BPVS with

BPVS	Variable	Coefficient of correlation 'r'
Vocabulary Age	Chronological Age	+ 0.24
Raw Score	Boehm Test of Basic Concepts (Raw Score)	+ 0.76
Raw Score	Sentence Comprehension Test (Raw Score)	+ 0.68
Vocabulary Age	Picture Arrangement Test (WISC) (Raw Score)	+ 0.68

other measures are given in the following table.

It is not surprising to note that there is no significant correlation between Vocabulary Age as on BPVS and Chronological Age among autistics. It is at the expected level only. What is more interesting is that language development takes place as a whole in the case of autistics. There is no clear cut divergence among different aspects of language development. Rather there is a significant moderate correlation between receptive vocabulary, understanding of basic concepts (Spatial Relations, Temporal Relations, Quantitative and Miscellaneous), sentence comprehension as well as use of language in logical thinking as in the case of picture arrangement sub-test of WISC. This finding is highly instructive. The earlier investigators (Bartak, Rutter and Cox, 1975; Lockyer and Rutter, 1970; Tymchuk, Simmoms and Neafsey, 1977; Wassing, 1965) found that autistics have difficulty performing both verbal and nonverbal tasks requiring sequencing skills. They also have difficulty conceptualising language (Rutter, 1978a, 1978b). Ohta (1987) objects that it is not clear what kinds of abnormalities exist in concept formation. He himself examined some studies which have shown that autistic children have difficulty in acquiring concepts of relationships. On the basis of the findings of those studies, Ohta (1987) infers that impairment in determination of relationships, such as comparisons and spatial relationships, may be a characteristic disorder of infantile autism.

The inference drawn by Ohta (1987) does not seem to be substantiated as there exists a significant correlation between raw scores on BPVS and that of Boehms Test of Basic Concepts which assesses relational concepts. That means those who have difficulty in receptive vocabulary have difficulty in relational concepts also. On the other hand if a child is good in receptive vocabulary, he will be good in relational concepts as well.

Investigators like Bartak, Rutter and Cox (1975); Lockyer and Rutter (1970); Tymchuk, Simmoms and Neafsey (1977); Wassing (1965) found characteristic performance pattern on the WISC by autistics. They observed that autistics have difficulty performing both verbal and nonverbal tasks requiring sequencing skills. Whereas Gillies (1965) found that the psychotics (autistics) did relatively better than the controls on the Object Assembly and Picture Arrangement of the WISC, Mair (1964) (cited in Mittler, 1968) reported significantly higher Block Design (WISC) scores in psychotics. Mittler (1968) interpreted that these tests require sequential ordering of stimuli rather than verbal mediation. However, in the study by Ramaa and Mittler (1991), significant correlation has been found between scores on picture arrangement and receptive vocabulary, which in turn is highly correlated with relational concepts, and sentence comprehension. Thus it is a wrong idea to consider that performance on Picture Arrangement does not require verbal mediation. Though it is classified under Performance Test, still it not only has perceptual-organization component, but is also loaded with verbal skills, like use of inner language. The poor performance noticed by some of the investigators on picture arrangement test (sequential test), thus can be attributed to language deficit, rather than to perceptual deficits.

The important implication is that a purposeful and deliberate attempt has to be made to develop inner language — receptive vocabulary, relational concepts, sentence pattern, and use of language for logical/sequential thinking among autistics. Development of inner language may contribute to success in academic performance, as it facilitates meaningfulness of the content to be learned by autistics.

CHAPTER 7

Summary: Picture of Autism Emerging from a Multidisciplinary Perspective

In the previous chapters an extensive review of different theories of autism has been made. Each theory seems to be successful in explaining some of the behavioural symptoms of autism. So they can be selectively synthesized in order to yield a more comprehensive and adequate picture than any one theory or set would do.

Investigators like Ornitz (1983) believe that there are two types of autism — primary and secondary. They differ mainly in the aetiological or associated factors but share common pathologies in neuropsychological, neuroanatomical and neurochemical aspects of development. These pathologies either in isolation or in combination lead to autism which is a unique behavioural syndrome. Since aetiologies or associated factors as well as resulting pathology are different, it is very difficult to give one single but adequate explanation to all the symptoms of autism. Moreover, many findings of research are tentatively accepted and they are yet to reach a conclusive state. So it will be too early to generalise the findings of research based on any one set of theoretical assumptions. Hence an attempt has been made below to give an integrative and harmonious but tentative explanation to different aspects of autistic syndrome.

First of all autism can be considered as a complex learning disorder in contrast to specific learning disorders like dyslexia and dyscalculia. While it is difficult to explain specific learning disorders, even today it would be extremely challenging to explain a complex learning disorder. So whatever attempt we make to draw the total picture of autism it remains incomplete and unsatisfactory. However, a beginning in sketching is necessary; more and more links and explanations can be added later on, suitable modifications can also be made where necessary.

The biogenic theories indicate three possible causative factors of autism namely genetic basis, presence of fragile-X and abnormalities in the neurobiological system, particularly brainstem pathology. However, it is hypothesised that damage at the brainstem level lead to dysfunction of higher centres of brain. There is a need to find out the aetiological factor(s) through different techniques. Early detection of conditions like fragile-X is helpful as the condition can be treated through folic acid; this may then be supplemented with early intervention programmes in the area of language and social skills. This might improve the behavioural adjustment and level of functioning among autistics.

The neurophysiological theories focus on certain functional defects as causes of autism. Altered immune response is one such functional defect. Some investigators suspect that this defect may be due to pre-exposure to certain antigens such as bacterial, viral or other material such as food or the environment. So avoidance of these antigens is necessary for preventing autism.

Metabolic error is also considered as an explanation for autism. According to this hypothesis autistic syndrome is considered as the result of a genetic peptidase deficiency, which causes peptide accumulation and further peptidase inhibition. As peptide overload is mainly of dietary origin, dietary treatment is essential. This can prepare the autistic individual for physiological or behavioural treatment.

The third defect which is considered to be a causal factor for autism is opioid excess. According to this hypothesis autistic children have a low desire for companionship, many of their eventual cognitive deficits may be secondary to their failure to learn social norms and cultural knowledge. This characteristic feature of autistics is attributed to excessive brain opioid activity. It is thought to constitutionally inhibit social motivation resulting in autistic aloofness. Opiate blocking agents such as naltrexone and naloxane are found to be effective in reducing the active symptoms of autism such as stereotypes, hyperactivity, self-injurious behaviours and aggressiveness and are effective in enhancing pro-social/behaviours among autistics.

The information processing deficit theories are included under psycho-physiological theories. According to these theories a confusion of sensory input combined with lack of language could result in a state of autism. In autistics there may be faulty sensory input, faulty transmission of the input, faulty filtration/selection of data, and/or difficulties in making comparison with "records" which may themselves be faulty. The process of filtration/selection of data is of particular importance to normal existence. The defect in this process leads to deficit in the habituation process. As a result, the individual is less effective in filtering out those stimuli which are significant from those which are not. It is hypothesised that this defect not only leads to cognitive difficulties but also to defects in emotional and social interpretations. Thus as per this theory defect in the filtration/selection of data is the fundamental problem in autism. This defect is attributed to higher concentration of peptides. So controlling the level of peptides forms the first step in treating autistics. This has to be followed by psycho-educational interventions.

All the pathology underlying autistic syndromes are not yet scientifically established. In this context what Shattock (1990) concluded seems to be more logical. According to him the current medical intervention strategies may not be considerably effective in overcoming the basic defects among autistics. It is possible that various Neuroanatomical and Neurophysiological abnormalities as well as conditions like Fragile-X syndrome may be correlated with each other. These kinds of correlative studies have to be conducted systematically with larger population, if possible causal relations have to be established among these diverse factors. Therefore till medical strategies become effective in either totally preventing, or eliminating complex learning disorders among autistics, these problems must be dealt with through psycho-educational intervention techniques. Therefore parallel studies have to be conducted in psychological and educational aspects also. The body of knowledge accumulated in these areas have to be carefully considered for helping individuals with autism.

The purely psychological theories deal with language deficits and social and pragmatic deficits among autistics. The language theory emphasises that language impairment is a major defect among autistics. Various attempts have been made to distinguish autistics from mentally retarded and dysphasics as far as language functioning is concerned. It was noticed that autistics exhibit certain unique deficits which are not found in the mentally retarded and dysphasics. On the basis of such observations Rutter (1983) concluded that autism is associated with both language abnormalities and cognitive deficits that are more severe, more widespread and somewhat different in pattern from those found in developmental 'dysphasia'. The two important characteristics of language among autistics are their relative failure to use language for social communication and abnormality in social interactions. So there is a need to understand the social impairments and the possible cognitive deficits that might underlie them, in autistics.

Many studies have been conducted to study the social and pragmatic deficits among autistics. The social impairment of autistics can be classified into three types — social aloofness, passive interaction, and active-but-odd interaction. It was noticed that the category to which any autistic child falls differs according to his/her age, gender, familiarity and characteristics of their playmates and other associates. The impairment also progresses developmentally from 'aloof' to 'passive' in social responsiveness, and from 'aloof' to 'passive' to 'odd' in rate of initiation of interaction. That means though there is change in the nature of social impairment it still persists. However, there are certain unimpaired areas in social understanding of autistic children. They are face recognition, mirror self-recognition, and perceptual role-taking. So an important task of psychological theories in the area of social impairment among autistics is to explain this kind of uneven profile.

Autistic children's speech is characterised by more egocentric remarks which reflect echolalia, self-repetition thinking aloud, and sometimes apparently purposeless remarks. According to Piaget's (1932) theory this excessive egocentric speech can be attributed to autistics' inability to cross beyond egocentricism. Thus autism may be considered to represent an immaturity of development.

Very interesting attempts have been made to explain social and pragmatic deficits among autistics. These explanations fall into different theoretical perspectives. The first set of theories are cognitive theories. Piaget's Two-Factor Theory was used extensively to explain most of the autistic syndromes.

The explanations given by Morgan (1986) on the basis of Piaget's Two-Factor Theory seems to be adequate with most of the crucial aspects relating to deviance in development of social relationships, abnormalities in communication, as well as restricted, repetitive and stereotyped patterns of behaviour among autistic individuals. However no attempt has been made to explain sensory deviation among them. Still this theory can be considered as the relatively most satisfactory theory for explaining autistic syndromes. But what biological explanation can be given to the observation that most of the autistics are normal in figurative aspect of cognitive development but deficient in operative aspect? Can we hypothesise that the centres of the brain which are dealing with these two aspects of development are different? If so, is it only those centres which deal with operative aspects are affected in a majority of the autistics? Are the aetiologies and resulting pathologies different for children who have deficiency in both figurative and operative aspects of cognitive development and those who are deficient only in the latter? Future research should try to answer questions like the above.

Another important theory for explaining the Social and Pragmatic deficits of autistics is meta-representation theory. The basic assumption of this theory is that meta-representation is a cognitive ability. It is essential in social skills which involve attributing mental states such as beliefs and desires to others. Since autistics have deficiency in meta-representational capacity — social skills which require it are deficient in them; whereas the social skills which do not require meta-representational capacity may be unimpaired in autism.

The theory of meta-representation also indirectly suggests that there is a cleavage in the cognitive development among autistics. As understood above, autistics may fail to cross beyond egocentricism. This may also be attributed to deficiency in the operative aspect of cognitive development among autistics.

Another point is, meta-representation theory tries to explain social and pragmatic deficits unidirectionally. In fact there is a circular relationship between meta-representational capacity and social and pragmatic deficits. The deficiency in one leads to deficiency in the other.

The above idea is supported indirectly by Affective theory. According to this theory by Habson, autism should be considered as a disorder of affective and social relations. This disorder in turn leads to cognitive and language disabilities. Thus both affective theory and meta-representational theory are complementary to each other.

The theory of inner language among autistics suggest that development of inner language is very poor among autistic children, and such a poverty forms an important feature among them. Various illustrations based on systematic observation are given to explain how deficiency in inner language affects the functioning capacity of autistics at different stages of development.

According to Wallace and Kauffman (1973) inner language is dependent upon the child's ability to: (i) establish imagery for sounds, words, concept, etc. and (ii) use the complex maze of skills needed in the logical thinking process. So development of concepts and logical thinking are essential for inner language development. The poverty in inner language among autistics can also be explained on the basis of Piaget's Two-Factor Theory. In young autistic children there is a delay even in figurative aspects of cognitive development. That is why autistic children fail to attain the concepts of common objects. Gradually these operations may emerge but the development of operations relating to operative aspects of cognitive development may either be arrested or delayed. The cognitive skills relating to figurative dimension are essential for performance on tasks relating to operative dimension. This is demonstrated in a study by Ramaa and Mittler (1991) where they found out significant positive moderate correlations between vocabulary development on the one hand and basic concepts (relational concepts — spatial, temporal and quantitative) and sentence comprehension, and ability to arrange pictures in logical sequence, on the other.

The important implication is that a purposeful and deliberate attempt has to be made to develop inner language among autistics. Development of inner language may enhance academic performance, as it facilitates meaningfulness of the content to be learnt by autistics. It also may enhance overall functioning among them.

Taking cognizance of the different theoretical perspectives, autism can be understood as follows. Autism is a complex learning disorder. It could be attributed to different defects at the biological level. These defects may affect certain physiological functions which in turn may affect the sensory inputs, mainly filtration/selection of sensory data. They may also reduce social desire among autistics. These two together reduce the interaction of autistic individuals with the environment. The reduced interaction hampers the cognitive, language, social and pragmatic development among autistics. As all these dimensions are correlated with each other, deficiency in one area leads to deficiency in other areas of development. Thus it yields an interaction model of development, that is, both inborn deficiency and environmental deprivation leads to autism.

The cleavage in cognitive development among autistics can be explained as due to defect or dysfunction of only those centres of brain which deal with operative aspect of cognitive development. Thus the level of autism depends upon the nature of aetiology and resulting pathophysiology. There is a need to establish links at all these levels.

Since many autistics have disability in processing sensory input the nature of such a disability has to be understood properly. The intervention programme must include correction of underlying dysfunction at the physiological level and psycho-educational programmes to enhance/improve the skills necessary for proper processing and sensory input. Underlying pathology for autistic aloofness should be corrected and social interaction has to be facilitated. The biological and/or physiological factors relating to cognitive deficits have to be determined. If possible they have to be corrected.

Along with this, deliberate attempts have to be made to enhance cognitive, language, social and pragmatic skills through psycho-educational intervention programmes. It is interesting to notice that though the research work relating to causal factors for autism are still in premature stage psycho-educational intervention programmes are being carried to foster the development of all the skills among autistics. Though there is considerable improvement among those autistics who are subjected to such programmes majority of them are still far below the normal level of functioning in all these skills. They do not reach mastery level. Moreover the programme should be intensive and they consume a lot of time and energy. In most of these cases it becomes a life long process and in some cases the improvement is negligible. When psycho-educational treatments are preceded by or supplemented with adequate medical intervention it may be possible to develop the essential skills among autistics without too much of taxing efforts. The trends of research in the medical field relating to autism reveal that such a day is not very far off.

Bibliography

American Psychiatric Association, *DSM-III Diagnostic and Statistical Manual of Mental Disorders* (3rd edn.), Washington, DC: American Psychiatric Association 1980.

American Psychiatric Association, *DSM-III-R Diagnostic and Statistical Manual of Mental Disorders* (revised), Washington, DC: American Psychiatric Association 1987.

American Psychiatric Association, *DSM-IV Diagnostic and Statistical Manual of Mental Disorders,* Washington, DC: American Psychiatric Association 1994.

Anthony, J. Low grade psychosis in childhood, *Proceedings of the London Conference for the Scientific Study of Mental Deficiency,* Vol. 2, B.W. Richards (ed.), May and Baker, London, 1962.

August, G.J., and Lockhart, L.H. *Familiar autism and the Fragile-X chromosome. Journal of Autism and Developmental Disorders,* 14, 197–204.

Bauman, M., Kemper, T.L. Histoanatomic observations of the brain in early infantile autism. *Neurology* 35, 866–874, 1985.

Baron-Cohen, Social and Pragmatic Deficits in Autism: Cognitive or Affective? *Journal of Autism and Developmental Disorders,* Vol. 18, No. 3, 1988.

Bartak, L., Rutter, M. and Cox, A comparative study of infantile autism and specific developmental receptive language disorder: I The Children British. *Journal of Psychiatry,* 126, 127–145, 1975.

Bates, E. Language in Context. New York: Academic Press, 1976.

Boucher, J. Articulation in early childhood autism. *Journal of Autistic and·Childhood*. Schizophrenia, 6, 297–302, 1976.

Bettelheim, B. *The Empty Fortress: Infantile Autism and the Birth of the Self*. London: Collier-Macmillan, 1967.

Carpenter, N.J. et al. Controlled six month study of folic acid therapy in boys with Fragile-X linked mental retardation. Paper presented at the 34th Annual Meeting of the American Society of Human Genetics, Norfolk, Virginia, November, 1983.

Campbell, M. et al. Naltrexone in Autistic children: An acute open dose range tolerance trial. *Journal of American Academy of Child and Adolescent Psychiatry*, 28, 200–206, 1989.

Caplan and Walker, Transformational Deficits in cognition of schizophrenic children, *Journal of Autism and Developmental Disorders*, Vol. 9, No. 2, 1979.

Churchill, D.W. Language: The Problem beyond Conditioning. In Rutter, M. and Schopler E. (eds.), *Autism: A Reappraisal of Concepts and Treatment*. New York: Plenum, 1978.

Cowman, P.A. Piaget, *With feeling*, New York, Holt, Rinehart, and Winston, 1978.

Clements John, *Severe Learning Disability and Psychological Handicap*, John Wiley and Sons Ltd., 1987.

Courchesne, E. et al. Abnormal Neuroanatomy in a Nonretarded person with Autism. *Arch. Neurol*. 44, 335–341, 1987.

Courchesne, E. et al. Hypoplasia of cerebellar vermal lobules VI and VII in autism, *New England Journal of Medicine*, 318, 1349–1354, 1988.

Creak, M. and Ini, S. Families of psychotic children. *Journal of Child Psychology and Psychiatry*, 1, 156–175, 1960.

Cunningham, M.A. A comparison of the language psychotic and nonpsychotic children who are mentally retarded. *Journal of Child Psychology and Psychiatry*, 9, 229–244, 1968.

Dahlgren, S.P. and Gillberg, C. Symptoms in the first two years of life; a preliminary population study of infantile autism. *European Archives of Psychiatry and Neurological Sciences*, 238, 169–174, 1989.

Demyer, M.K. Motor, perceptual motor and intellectual disabilities of Autistic children. In Wing, L. (ed.) *Early Childhood Autism*, Pergamon Press, 1976.

Dennet, D. Brainstorms: *Philosophical essays of mind and Psychology*, Harvester Press, 1978.

Ekman, G. et al. Children with Infantile Autism Investigated by Magnetic Resonance Imaging, *Experimental Biology and the Autism Syndrome,* Collection of the papers from the conference. University of Durham, March 29–31, 1989.

Engeland, V.H. Information Processing Deficits in Early Infantile Autism: A psychophysiological Approach. *Experimental Biology and the Autistic Syndromes,* Collection of papers from the Conference, University of Durham, March 29–31, 1949.

Fernell, E., Gillberg, C. and Von Wendt, L. Autistic symptoms in children with infantile hydrocephalus. *Acta Paediatricia Scandinavica,* 1990.

Gaffrey, G.R., Tsai, L.Y. Brief Report: Magnetic Resonance Imaging of High Level Autism. *Journal of Autism and Developmental Disorders,* 17(3), 433–438, 1987.

Gaffrey, G.R. et al. Morphological evidence for brainstem involvement in infantile Autism, *Biological Psychiatry,* 24, 578–586, 1988.

Gillberg, C. Asperger syndrome in 23 Swedish children: A clinical study. *Developmental Medicine and Child Neurology,* 31, 520–531.

Gillberg, C. Autism and Pervasive Developmental Disorders, *Journal of Child Psychology and Psychiatry,* Vol. 31, No. 1, 99–119, 1990

Gillberg, I.C. and Gillberg, C. Asperger syndrome-some epidemiological considerations: research note. *Journal of Childpsychology and Psychiatry,* 30, 631–638.

Gillberg Christopher, Ohlson Vivi-Ann et al. Monozygotic Female twins with Autism and the Fragile-X Syndrome (AFRAX), *Journal of Child Psychology and Psychiatry,* Vol. 29, No. 4, pp. 447, 451, 1988.

Gillberg, C. and Steffenlurg, S. Outcome and prognostic factors in infantile autism and similar conditions. *Journal of Autism and Developmental Disorders,* 17, 271–285, 1987.

Gillies, S. Some abilities of Psychotic Children and Subnormal Controls. *Journal of Mental Deficiency Research,* 9, 89–101, 1965.

Gustavson et al. Effect of folic acid treatment in the fragile-X syndrome, *Clinical Genetics,* 27, 463–467, 1985.

Herold, S. et al. Cerebral blood flow and metabolism of oxygen and glucose in young autistic adults, *Psychological Medicine,* 18, 823–831, 1988.

Herman, B. et al. Naltexone decreases self-injurious behaviour. *Annals of Neurology*, 22, 550–552.

Hermelin, B.A. and O. Connor. N. *Psychological Experiments with Autistic Children*, Oxford, 1970.

Hermelin B. Coding and the sense modalities. In Wing, L. (ed.) *Early Childhood Autism*, Pergamon Press, 1976.

Hermelin, B. Recent Experimental Research. In Aspects of Autism, Mittler, P.J. London: *British Psychological Society*, 1968.

Israngkun, P.P. et al. *Neurochem Pathology*, 5, 51–70, 1986.

James, A.L. and Barry, R.J. A review of psychophysiology in early onset psychosis, *Schizophrenia Bulletin*, 6(3), 1980.

Johnson-Laird, *Mental Models*, Cambridge, England: Cambridge University Press, 1983.

Kanner, Autistic Disturbances of affective contact, *Nervous Child*, 2, 217–250, 1943.

Leboyer, M.M., Bouvard, M. and Dugas, M. Effects of naltrexone on infantile autism. *The Lancet*, 715.

Lejeune, J. Is the fragile-X syndrome amenable to treatment? *The Lancet*, 30 January, 273–274, 1982.

Leslie, A.M. Pretence and Representation; *The Origins of Theory of Mind, Psychological Review*, 94, 412–426.

Lockyer, L., and Rutter, M. A five to fifteen year follow-up study of infantile psychosis. III. Psychological Aspects. *British Journal of Psychiatry*, 115, 865–882, 1970.

Lord, C. Peer relations in autism. In F.J. Morrison, C. Lord and D.P. Keating (ed.) *Applied Developmental Psychology*, Vol. I, pp. 165–229, New York: Academic Press, 1984.

Lotter V. Epidemiology of autistic conditions in young children, II, Some characteristics of the parents and children. *Social Psychiatry*, 1, 163–173, 1967.

Luria, A.R. *The Role of Speech in the Regulation of Normal and Abnormal Behaviour*, London: Pergamon Press, 1961.

Markowitz, P.I. Autism in a child with congenital cytomegalovirus infection, *Journal of Autism and Developmental Disorders*, 13, 249–253, 1983.

Mittler, P.J. (ed.) Aspects of Autism — Some Approaches to Childhood Psychoses, London, *British Psychological Society*, 1968.

Mittler, P. and Ward, J. The use of the Illinois Test of Psycholinguistic Abilities on British Four-Year-Old Children: A Normative and Factorial Study, *British Journal of Psychology*, 1970.

Morgan, B. Sam Autism and Piagete's Theory: Are the two compatible? *Journal of Autism and Developmental Disorders,* Vol. 16, No. 4, 1986.

Ohman, A. The orientation response, attention and learning: An information processing perspective. In H.D. Kimmel, E.H. Van Olst and J.F. Orlebeke (ed.): *The Orienting Reflex in Humans,* Hillsdale New Jersey: Lawrence Erlbaum Ass. 1980.

Ohta, M. Cognitive Disorders of Infantile Autism: A Study Employing the WISC, Spatial Relationship, Conceptualisation and Gesture Imitations, *Journal of Autism and Developmental Disorders,* Vol. 17, No. 1, 1987.

Ornitz, E.M. Childhood autism. A disorder of sensory and motor integration. In M. Rutter (ed.). *Infantile Autism: Concepts, Characteristics and Treatment,* 50–68, London: Churchill-Livingstone, 1971.

Ornitz, E.M. The modulation of sensory input and motor output in autistic children, *Journal of Autism and Developmental Disorders,* 10, 347–360, 1969.

Ornitz, E.M. Vestibular dysfunction in schizophrenia and childhood autism, *Comprehensive Psychiatry,* 11, 159–173, 1970.

Ornitz, E.M. Neurophysiology of infantile autism. *Journal of the American Academy of Child and Adolescent Psychiatry,* 24, 251–262, 1985.

Ornitz, E.M. Sensory modulation and directed attention in autism. Paper read at the World Federation of Societies of Biological Psychiatry Congress, Jerusalem, April, 1969.

Panskeep, J.A. Neurochemical theory of Autism. *Trends in Neuroscience,* 2, 174–177, 1979.

Panskeep, J. Brain Opioids: A Neurochemical substrate for Narcotic and Social Dependence. *In Progress in Theory in Psychopharmacology.* S. Cooper (ed.) London: Academic Press, 149–175, 1981.

Panskeep, J., Lensing, P. The opioid excess theory of Autism: Theoretical and Empirical Bases, Experimental Biology and the Autism Syndromes, University of Durham, Collection of the papers from the conference, March 29–31, 1989.

Panskeep, J. and Sahlay, T. Possible brain opioid involvement in disrupted social intent and language development of autism. *In: Neurobiological Issues in Autism,* E. Schopler and G. Mesibov (ed.), Plenum Press, New York, 357–373.

Panskeep, J. et al. Endogenous opioids and social behaviour, *Neuroscience and Biobehavioural Reviews*, 4, 473–487, 1980.

Panskeep, J. et al. Opiates and play Dominance in Juvenile Rats. *Behavioural Neuroscience*, 99, 441-453, 1985.

Panskeep, J. et al. Neural and Neurochemical control of the separation distress call. In J.D. Newman (ed.). *The Physiological Control of Mammalian Vocalizations*. Plenum Press, 263–300, 1988.

Piaget, J. *The Language and Thought of the Child*, London; Routledge and Kegan Paul, 1932.

Pollack, M. Comparison of childhood, adolescent and adult Schizophrenics, *Arch. Gen. Psychiat.*, 2, 652–660, 1960.

Pylyshyn, When is attribution of beliefs justified? *Behavioural and Brain Sciences*, I, 592–593.

Ramaa and Mittler, Inner Language among Verbal Autistic Children. Accepted for publication in *Journal of All India Institute of Speech and Hearing*, Mysore, 1997.

Reiichelt et al. Autistic Syndromes; Possible Etiology and Treatment, Experimental Biology and the Autistic Syndromes, University of Durham, Collection of the papers from the Conference, March 29–31, 1989.

Reiss, A.L. Correspondence. *The New England Journal of Medicine*, 319(17); 1152–1153, 1988.

Ritvo, E.R. et al. Lower Purkinje Cell counts in the cerebella of four autistic subjects; initial findings of the VCLA-NSAC autopsy research report. *American Journal of Psychiatry*, 143, 862–866, 1986.

Ricks, D.M. and Wing, L. Language, communication and the use of symbols. In Wing, L. (ed.) *Early Childhood Autism*, Pergamon Press, 1976.

Rimland, B. *Infantile Autism* New York: Appleton-Century-Crafts, 1964.

Rimland, B. On the objective diagnosis of infantile autism. *Acta Paedopsychiatrica*, 35, 146–160, 1966.

Rowell, F.J. The Immune System and Autism; Introduction. Experimental Biology and the autistic Syndromes, University of Durham, Collection of the papers from the Conference, March 29-31, 1989.

Rutter, M. Language Disorder and Infantile Autism. In Rutter, M. and Schopler (eds.), *Autism: A Reappraisal of Concepts and Treatment*, New York: Plenum, 1978a.

Rutter, M. Diagnosis and Definition. In Rutter, M. and Schopler (eds.), *Autism: A Reappraisal of Concepts and Treatment*, New York: Plenum, 1978b.

Rutter, M. Language, Cognition and Autism. In: Katzman (ed.), *Congenital and Acquired Cognitive Disorders*, 247–264, New York.

Rutter, M. Cognitive Deficits in the Pathogenesis of Autism, *Journal of Child Psychology and Psychiatry*, Vol. 24, No. 4, 513–531, 1983.

Rutter, M. and Schopler, E. Autism and Pervasive Developmental Disorders: Concepts and Issues, *Journal of Autism and Developmental Disorders*, Vol. 17, No. 2, 159–186, 1987.

Rutter, M. Psychotic disorders in early childhood. In: *Recent Developments in Schizophrenia;* A Symposium. Ed. Copper, A. J. and Walk, A. London; RMPA, 1967.

Rutter, M. Concepts of Autism in Mittler, P.J. (ed.). Aspects of Autism some Approaches to Childhoodpsychoses, London: *British Psychological Society*, 1968.

Rutter, M. Prognosis. In: Wing, J.K. (ed.) *Early Childhood Autism: Clinical, Educational and Social Aspects*. London: Pergamon, 1966.

Rutter, M. Autistic Children; Infancy to Adulthood: *Semin Psychiat*, 2, 435–450, 1970.

Sahley, T.L. and Panskeep, J. Brain opioids and Autism; An updated Analysis of possible Linkages. *Journal of Autism and Developmental Disorders*, 201–216, 1987.

Shattok, P. In: Aspects of Autism; Biological Research, Wing, L. (ed.), Gaskell/The National Autistic Society, 11-18, 1988.

Shattock, P. The possible neuroregulatory role of peptides in autism, Experimental Biology and the Autistic Syndromes, Collection of papers from the Conference, University of Durham, March 29-31, 1989.

Shattock, P. Some Implications of Basic Physiological Research for the behaviour and treatment of people with Autism, experimental Psychology and the Autistic Syndromes, Collection of papers from the conference, University of Durham, April 18–20, 1990.

Sigman, M. and Ungerer, J.A. Cognitive and language skills in autistic, mentally retarded and normal children, *Developmental Psychology*, 20, 293–302, 1984.

Stubbs, E.G. Autistic children exhibit undetectable hemagglutination-inhibition antibody titres despite previous rubella vaccination. *J. Autism and Childhood Schizophrenia*, 6, 269–274, 1976.

Stubbs. E.G. Autistic Symptoms in a child with congenital cytomegalovirus infection, *Journal of Autism and Childhood Schizophrenia*, 8, 37–43, 1978.

Stubbs, E.G., Ash, E., and Williams, C.P.S. Autism and Congenital Cytomegalovirus, *Journal of Autism and Developmental Disorders*, 7, 49–55, 1984.

Stubbs, E.G. *In: aspects of Autism: Biological Research*, ed. Lorna Wing, Gaskell. The National Autistic Society, 91–101, 1988.

Tantam, D. Annotation; Asperger's Syndrome. *Journal of Child Psychology and Psychiatry*, 29, 245–255, 1988.

The Association of Head Teachers of Autistic Children and Adults (1985), The Special Curricular Needs of Autistic Children, U.K.

Todd, R.D., and Ciaranello, R.D. Demonstration of inter and intraspecies differences in serotonim binding sites by antibodies from an autistic child, *Proc. Natt. Acrd. Sci. USA*, 82, 612–616, 1985.

Tymchuk, A.J., Simmons, J.A. and Neafsey, S. Intellectual Characteristics of Adolescent Childhood Psychotics with High Verbal Ability. *Journal of Mental Deficiency Research*, 21, 133–138, 1977.

Uta Frith. *Autism Explaining the Enigma*, Basil Blackwell, 1989.

Vythilingam, Meena. Pervasive Developmental Disorder — An Exploratory Study, Thesis submitted for M.D. Degree (Unpublished), Bangalore University, 1991.

Wahlstrom, J., Gillberg, C., Gustavson, K.G. and Holmgren, G. Infantile autism and the fragile-X syndrome. A Swedish Population multicenter study. *American Journal of Medical Genetics*, 23, 403–408, 1986.

Warren, R.P., Foster, A., Margartten, N.C. et al. Immune abnormalities in patients with autism. *Journal of Autism and Developmental Disorders*, 16, 189–197, 1986.

Wassing, H.E. Cognitive functioning in early infantile autism: An examination of four cases by means of the Wechsler intelligence scale for children. *Acta Paedopsychiatrica*, 32, 122–135.

Weizman, A., Weizman, R. et al. Abnormal immune response to brain tissue antigen in the syndrome of autism. *American Journal of Psychiatry*, 139, 1462–1465, 1982.

Wing, L. Epidemiology and Theories of Aetiology. In Wing, L. (ed.) *Early Childhood Autism*, Pergamon Press, 1976.

Wing, L. *Asperger syndrome: A clinical account, psychological medicine*, 11, 115–129, 1981.

Wing, L. and Gould, J. Severe impairment of social interaction and associated abnormalities in children; epidemiology and classification. *Journal of Autism and Development Disorders*, 9, 129–137, 1979.

Wing, L. and Gould, J. Severe impairment of social interaction and associated abnormalities in children; epidemiology and classification. *Journal of Autism and Development Disorders*, 9, 11–29, 1979.

World Health Organisation, ICD-10; Draft of Chapter V, Categories F00-F99 mental, behavioural and developmental disorders. Geneva; World Health Organisation, 1992.